COGNITIVE AND BEHAVIORAL CHARACTERISTICS OF CHILDREN WITH LEARNING DISABILITIES

COGNITIVE AND BEHAVIORAL CHARACTERISTICS OF CHILDREN WITH LEARNING DISABILITIES

EDITED BY

Joseph K. Torgesen

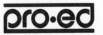

8700 Shoal Creek Boulevard
Austin, Texas 78758

The Austin Research Symposium Series
Funded by The Donald D. Hammill Foundation

Series Editor: J. Lee Wiederholt

Contents of this book were previously published in the
Journal of Learning Disabilities.

Printed in the United States of America

Library of Congress Cataloging-in-Publication Data

Cognitive and behavioral characteristics of children with learning
   disabilities / edited by Joseph K. Torgesen.
      p. cm.—(The Austin research symposium series)
   Proceedings of a research symposium held in Austin, Tex., Mar.
25–26, 1988.
   "Contents of this book were previously published in the Journal of
learning disabilities"—T.p. verso.
   Includes indexes.
   ISBN 0-89079-207-0
   1. Learning disabilities—Congresses. 2. Cognition disorders in
children—Congresses. 3. Learning disabled children—Psychology—
Congresses. 4. Dyslexia—Congresses. I. Torgesen, Joseph K.
II. Journal of learning disabilities. III. Series.
LC4704.C6 1990
371.9—dc20   90-10243
                                                 CIP

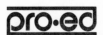

8700 Shoal Creek Boulevard
Austin, Texas 78758

10 9 8 7 6 5 4 3 2 1   90 91 92 93 94 95

Foreword

In the spring of 1988, The Donald D. Hammill Foundation sponsored the Austin Invitational Research Symposium. The topic of this particular symposium was the cognitive and behavioral characteristics of children with learning disabilities. The chapters contained in this book are the direct outgrowth of the discussions and contributions of the researchers and scholars who were invited to participate. The contents of this volume provide a rich, fascinating context for understanding this diverse and complex special population.

The trustees of the Foundation express their sincere appreciation to Professor Joseph K. Torgesen. Dr. Torgesen is on the faculty of the Department of Psychology at Florida State University. He pursued his graduate education in developmental and clinical psychology at Brigham Young University and the University of Michigan. The conceptualization of this symposium, the selection of the participating scholars, and the editing of the chapters herein we owe to his capable leadership.

J. Lee Wiederholt
Trustee
The Donald D. Hammill Foundation

vii

Preface

I have felt for some time that researchers studying learning disabilities need more opportunities to discuss each other's work in an atmosphere of openness and informality. At the typical large research meetings, there is never enough time for anything but a brief exchange that almost always begs for follow-up question and comment. Of course, a lot of discussion can occur one-on-one after a session or over dinner, but many who might profit from such discussions are not present. We need to have more small meetings, where participants have a better chance to get to know one another. Such opportunities can often lead to very productive collaborative relationships.

For these reasons, I was very pleased when The Donald D. Hammill Foundation agreed to fund a research symposium that would allow the intense interaction among participants we so often miss at larger meetings. We invited eight active researchers to present their work over 2 days of sessions. The meetings were informal, the number of observers was limited, and a big horseshoe table allowed us to face one another during discussions. Not only did we have ample opportunity to discuss each other's work, but we also enjoyed a very pleasant several days together in beautiful surroundings.

As one of the participants, I took a number of useful new ideas away from the symposium, and I know that others did as well. Although I have not attempted to distill the actual discussion from the symposium in this book, the chapters in it accurately reflect the content that we considered. I have tried to convey the main themes of the symposium, as well as points of consensus and disagreement, in my introductory and closing comments. I want to express my gratitude to the Hammill Foundation for making the symposium possible and to each of the participants for their work toward making it a success.

Joseph K. Torgesen

1. Introduction

JOSEPH K. TORGESEN

The most important goal of the symposium from which the chapters in this volume were taken was to facilitate communication of scientific information about learning disabilities at two levels. First, the symposium was structured with an emphasis on group discussion of the research that was presented. This extended opportunity for discussion was provided so that those in attendance would have more than the usual opportunities to affect one another's work through their comments and questions. A second, and much broader, level of communication is provided by publication of the papers presented at the symposium. Authors were asked to present their work in a manner that would not only contribute to the scientific knowledge base, but would also help readers to understand its implications for applied work with children with learning disabilities (LD). It is my task in this introduction to provide an overview of the presentations and to discuss the themes that emerged during the symposium. In a concluding chapter, I comment on the points about which there was consensus, the issues on which there was some disagreement, and the questions that clearly need further research.

The title of the symposium was "The Cognitive and Behavioral Characteristics of Children with Learning Disabilities." The word *cognitive* was meant to invite discussion of information processing skills that are usually not directly observable, but that can be verified and tested in the process of experimentation. Processing skills in this sense can be thought of as mental behaviors that must be performed in order

1

to successfully accomplish many academic, social, or intellectual tasks. Examples of such processing activities might include coding information for storage in working memory, comparing incoming information with the contents of long-term memory to check for similarities and discrepancies, and selecting an appropriate strategy to enhance performance on a task. By the term *behavioral*, we mean aspects of a child's behavior that are directly observable. Examples of such behaviors might include rate of problem solution, persistence on tasks, question asking, and specific off-task and on-task behaviors. Information about these types of behaviors is usually obtained by direct observational coding, or through parent and teacher rating forms.

The symposium focused on both cognitive and behavioral characteristics because both kinds of attributes are relevant to understanding the academic and social learning problems of children with learning disabilities. In addition, recent research (as well as long-standing clinical lore) suggests that the cognitive and behavioral characteristics of these children are not independent from one another. That is, specific cognitive difficulties can lead to, or often coexist with, a range of behavioral difficulties. Thus a child who initially fails in reading because of a specific processing deficit may eventually exhibit a range of maladaptive classroom behaviors developed as a result of early and chronic failure. Although traditional conceptualizations exclude behavioral difficulties as a primary *cause* of learning disabilities, there can be little doubt that these children's behavioral difficulties frequently do interfere with their ability to learn in school.

One of the themes that emerged early and persisted throughout the symposium was the issue of specificity. In Chapter 2, Keith Stanovich asks the question of specificity in terms of differences between "garden-variety" poor readers and children who are labeled as reading disabled or dyslexic. Garden-variety poor readers are children who have difficulties learning to read, but who are not identified as specifically impaired in reading. Stanovich presents data to show that these children suffer a relatively broad developmental lag in many different cognitive skills. In other words, their reading difficulties occur in the context of *general* learning difficulties that affect performance on many different kinds of tasks. Using his data on garden-variety poor readers as a foundation, Stanovich then draws on the work of other investigators to present a general model that helps us understand the reading problems of both the garden-variety and specific, or dyslexic, types of poor readers. This model has important implications for assessment and diagnostic practices, because it also helps us to understand more about the relationships between the two types of reading failure.

Although Stanovich's model clearly illustrates the important differences between garden-variety and dyslexic poor readers, it also proposes that deficits in phonological processing underlie the essential reading difficulties of most children of both types. In fact, a second theme that emerged during the symposium concerned the importance of phonological processing difficulties in explaining many of the reading difficulties of learning disabled children. Phonological processing refers to the use of phonological information (the sounds of speech) in processing written and oral language. Phonological processing deficits are manifest on tasks that require children to make explicit reports about the phonological structure of words, to efficiently code (or represent) the phonological features of words in short-term memory, and to rapidly access phonological information that is stored in long-term memory.

In Chapter 3, I present information about a special subgroup of learning disabled children who have extreme difficulties using phonological codes to store information in short-term memory. Children in this subgroup (which comprises about 15% to 20% of school identified learning disabled children) have special difficulties on any task that requires verbatim retention of verbal information over brief periods of time. My research has focused partially on the way in which phonological coding deficits affect performance on complex tasks; one of the tasks that is most dramatically affected by deficits in this area is ability to apply phonological information in decoding print.

Virginia Mann and colleagues also present information concerning the phonological processing difficulties of disabled readers. Much of her recent work has investigated the ways in which a core deficit in phonological processing (specifically, storage of phonological information in short-term memory) can affect performance on other language tasks. The central question has been whether oral language comprehension deficits of poor readers can be explained by their difficulties in storing information about specific words in sentences. In the two studies she reports in her chapter, she tests the specific proposition that children with reading disabilities may frequently miss the meaning of sentences because they do not accurately remember specific features of the rhythm, pitch, and emphasis used by the speaker to communicate meaning. Mann's work has relatively clear implications for the ways in which teachers should speak to many children with reading disabilities.

A third theme that emerged in several of the presentations concerned the diversity of children who are labeled learning disabled. In Chapter 2, Stanovich introduces the concept of diversity by showing how the pattern of cognitive skills and deficits defining severe reading disability might be continuously variable across children. The continuous, multidimensional variability that is part of his model helps us to understand why it has proven so difficult to identify a limited number of homogeneous subtypes in the learning disabled population. Rebecca Felton and Frank Wood present data that provide concrete evidence of diversity among children with learning disorders. Their research focuses on the differences between children with attention deficit disorder and those with reading disabilities, as well as the extent of overlap between the two categories. Using data from their extensive longitudinal project in North Carolina, they are able to document that these two disorders are associated with very different patterns of cognitive deficit.

The research reported by James McKinney focuses on several important questions concerning variability among children with learning disabilities. The most obvious result of his research has been the classification of school identified children into subtypes on the basis of their classroom behaviors. This effort documents the substantial variability among these children, with some subtypes showing essentially normal patterns of behavior and others exhibiting various kinds of maladaptive behavior. Another important contribution from this research has been evidence that the behavioral subtypes show different patterns of school achievement.

Rather than documenting diversity among children with learning disorders, Dale Schunk has been concerned with a careful analysis of one particular pattern of maladaptive behavior that is characteristic of many children who fail in school. Using the concept of self-efficacy as his central focus, he has shown that children's attitudes about their own abilities can have very important effects on the way they approach school tasks. Equally important, he has shown that it is possible to manipulate children's beliefs about themselves in a way that has a positive effect on their learning behavior.

The problems discussed by Dale Schunk are not specific to children identified as learning disabled, but are characteristic of many types of poor learners. Stephen Ceci and Jacquelyn Baker's chapter suggests another way that children with learning disabilities may be similar to children in other categories of poor learning. Drawing on his own research on semantic memory and problem solving in learning disabilities, he suggests that many of the performance problems of children with learning disabilities result from lack of specific types of knowledge rather than basic processing disabilities. This position is consistent with recent work in the field of cognitive psychology that has pointed to the central role of domain-specific knowledge in accounting for expert behavior on many tasks. It is an important perspective for the field of learning disabilities because it explains how deficits in a child's knowledge base can produce patterns of poor learning or performance that might be mistaken for lack of ability.

Chapter 9, by Joseph Campione, is different from the others in that it does not focus on documenting any particular characteristics of children with learning disorders. Rather, it discusses methods of assessing these characteristics in a way that can provide educationally useful information. It is helpful as a concluding chapter because it suggests ways of moving from research-based descriptions of these children as a whole (or in subgroups) to useful descriptions of individual children within specific educational settings. At the heart of Campione's discussion is an evaluation of the relative merits of assessing general versus domain-specific skills and knowledge for a range of educational purposes. He also reports on techniques of individual assessment that represent important alternatives to the standard psychometric evaluations that are often applied to children with learning disabilities.

As a final note, it must be recognized that the work of many important researchers studying the cognitive and behavioral characteristics associated with learning disabilities was not covered in this symposium. The chapters in this book should be taken as *examples* of some of the excellent work in this area, but they are clearly not comprehensive in their coverage. We hope that future symposiums will be able to extend our coverage to other important topics in a way that will contribute systematically to the creation of a sound knowledge base not only about the range of learning disorders themselves, but also about methods that can be used to treat them.

2. Explaining the Differences Between the Dyslexic and the Garden-Variety Poor Reader: The Phonological-Core Variable-Difference Model

KEITH E. STANOVICH

The field of learning disabilities (LD) is contentious, and it has a checkered history. It is commonplace to bemoan the state of confusion and disagreement in the field. Here, however, I wish to focus on a positive trend that is discernible in current research. There has recently been an increasing recognition that the field in some sense "got ahead of itself," that educational practice simply "took off" before a thorough investigation of certain foundational assumptions had been carried out. Thus, much recent research has a "get back to basics" feel to it, as researchers double back to retrace crucial empirical and theoretical steps that were skipped during the mad rush to implement what we now know were nascent hypotheses rather than established empirical facts.

The signs that the field is making an attempt to establish itself on a firmer foundation are numerous. The National Institute of Child Health and Development (NICHD) is supporting long overdue large-scale epidemiological and subtype investigations. The statistical and psychometric complexities of defining disabilities on the basis of behavioral and cognitive discrepancies are becoming more widely understood and are beginning to affect practice (McKinney, 1987; Reynolds, 1985).

The development I would like to focus on here is the recent flurry of work that goes back to the most critical foundational assumption underlying the learning disability concept: the concept of qualitative differences in cognitive/behavioral characteristics. I will confine the remaining discussion to reading disability—the most prevalent type of learning disability and also my particular area of expertise.

From the beginning, what has fueled both theoretical interest in dyslexia (and/or reading disability, specific reading retardation, etc.; the terms are used interchangeably here) and has justified differential educational treatment has been the assumption that the reading difficulties of the dyslexic stem from problems different from those characterizing the "garden-variety" poor reader (to use Gough & Tunmer's, 1986, term); or, alternatively, the assumption that if reading difficulties stem from the same factors, the degree of severity is so extreme for the dyslexic that it constitutes, in effect, a qualitative difference.

I should mention as an aside that I view the interminable semantic debates in developmental psychology over what constitutes a qualitative as opposed to a quantitative difference as utterly futile and scientifically useless. Alternative terms would do equally well and probably would not trigger what are essentially linguistic debates. Nevertheless, I use the terms for convenience, ease of communication, and to make clear the connections with previous research.

What *is* important is the experimental contrasts that have operationalized the idea of qualitative difference and/or differential causation in the literature. This operationalization has been dominated by two different designs. One is the reading-level match design, where an older group of dyslexic children is matched on reading level with a younger group of nondyslexic children. The cognitive characteristics and reading subskills of the two groups are then compared. The logic here is fairly straightforward. If the reading subskills and cognitive characteristics of the two groups do not match, then it would seem that they are arriving at their similar reading levels via different routes, and this would support the idea of differential causation. In contrast, if the reading subskill profiles of the two groups are identical, this would seem to undermine the rationale for the differential educational treatment of dyslexic children and for their theoretical differentiation. If dyslexic children are reading just like any other child who happens to be at their reading level, and are using the same cognitive skills to do so, why should we consider their reading behavior to be so special?

The second major design—one pertinent not only to theoretical issues but also the educational politics of LD—is to compare dyslexic children with children of the same age who are reading at the same level, but who are not labeled dyslexic. (Adapting the terminology of

Gough & Tunmer, 1986, this design will be termed the "garden-variety control" design.) Again, the inferences drawn are relatively straight-forward. If the reading subskills and cognitive characteristics of the two groups do not match, then it would seem that the two groups are arriving at their similar reading levels via different routes. In contrast, if the reading subskill profiles of the two groups are identical, this would certainly undermine the rationale for the differential educa-tional treatment of dyslexic children and would make dyslexic children considerably less interesting theoretically. As Fredman and Stevenson (1988) state, if "there is no clear distinction between the groups in terms of how they read, then the practice of identifying a special group of poor readers for special attention may no longer be necessary" (p. 105).

Unfortunately, the results of research employing both of these designs have been inconsistent. Empirically, there are reading-level match studies that have revealed similar processing profiles (Beech & Harding, 1984; Treiman & Hirsh-Pasek, 1985) and those that have identified differences (Baddeley, Ellis, Miles, & Lewis, 1982; Bradley & Bryant, 1978; Kochnower, Richardson, & DiBenedetto, 1983; Olson, Kliegl, Davidson, & Foltz, 1985; Snowling, 1980; Snowling, Stackhouse, & Rack, 1986). Similarly, garden-variety comparisons have supported qualitative similarity (Fredman & Stevenson, 1988; Taylor, Satz, & Friel, 1979) and difference (Jorm, Share, Maclean, & Matthews, 1986; Rutter & Yule, 1975; Silva, McGee, & Williams, 1985).

The mixed results have troubled many in the field because they relate to some of the foundational assumptions of the concept of dyslexia as it is used in both research investigations and in educational practice. Indeed, these unresolved issues have provoked Andrew Ellis (1985) to ask, in an emperor-has-no-clothes fashion, "Is it worth studying dyslexia?" (p. 199); and to further press the point:

> Does applying all the exclusionary tests discussed earlier to a group of poor readers in order to obtain a sample of high-grade, refined dyslexics actually yield a sample whose reading problems are qualitatively different from those of non-dyslexic subjects? Surprisingly this question seems to have received hardly any attention at all. . . . No one, it seems, has ever shown that the initial laborious screening is necessary in the sense that it produces a population of individuais whose reading characteristics are different from the great mass of poor readers. (pp. 199–200)

Ellis's use of the word "surprisingly" alludes to the point mentioned earlier—that the field of learning disabilities expanded and grew in virtual absence of the critical data needed to test its foundational assumptions. This situation has only recently begun to be remedied by researchers employing the two designs that I described above.

Unfortunately, as was mentioned, the results have been somewhat equivocal. It has not always been possible to differentiate the performance of dyslexic children from garden-variety poor readers or from younger reading-level controls. Thus, the field still invites skeptical questioning like that of Ellis, and challenges such as,

> It may be timely to formulate a concept of reading disability which is independent of any consideration of IQ. Unless it can be shown to have some predictive value for the nature of treatment or treatment outcome, considerations of IQ should be discarded in discussions of reading difficulties. (Share, McGee, & Silva, in press, p. 12)

or,

> If the dyslexic readers differ from poor readers along the same dimensions that differentiate poor readers from good, it cannot be concluded that the dyslexic readers' performance is due to decoding processes specific to this group. Hence the results fail to provide evidence for the kind of qualitative differences between groups entailed by the standard view. ... If a term is to be reserved for those children who perform at the lowest end of the continuum, we suggest that it be something other than "dyslexic" or "reading disabled," which carry other connotations. Perhaps simply "very poor readers" would do. (Seidenberg, Bruck, Fornarolo, & Backman, 1986, pp. 79–80)

THE DEVELOPMENTAL LAG MODEL

One notable theoretical attempt to salvage the dyslexia concept has been the characterization of reading disabled children as not qualitatively different, but as suffering from a developmental lag in reading-related cognitive processes. The developmental lag notion has a venerable history in the psychology of mental retardation (see Zigler, 1969). Its theoretical importance in the LD literature resides in the fact that, unlike the deficit models that emphasize qualititative difference, lag models predict that when older disabled and younger nondisabled children are matched on reading level, their performance should not differ on any cognitive tasks causally related to reading (see Fletcher, 1981). Thus, at least some of the results that are problematic for those wishing to distinguish dyslexic children (e.g., the similarities in some reading-level control studies) are accommodated by the developmental lag theory.

However, there are several problems involved in conceptualizing and testing the lag notion. For example, predictions derived from the lag hypothesis depend critically on how the matching on reading level is done. It is somewhat surprising to find that researchers have been quite inconsistent in specifying exactly what "reading level" refers to in this literature or, for that matter, in the research employing garden-variety controls. Specifically, some investigations have matched children with reading comprehension tests (e.g., Bruck, 1988; Seidenberg, Bruck, Fornarolo, & Backman, 1985), while others have matched the children on word recognition skills (e.g., Olson et al., 1985; Treiman & Hirsh-Pasek, 1985). And finally, some have matched children using a composite of both word recognition and reading comprehension (Bloom, Wagner, Reskin, & Bergman, 1980; Jorm et al., 1986). Unfortunately, all of these investigations have been referred to as reading-level (RL) match studies, thus substantially increasing the difficulty of integrating the research findings in this area. It has been insufficiently recognized that the results and interpretation of an RL-match design may vary depending upon whether the matching is done with a comprehension test or with a word recognition test. We have suggested (Stanovich, Nathan, & Zolman, 1988) that future investigators refer to their designs as either decoding-level matches or comprehension-level matches.

The necessity of differentiating decoding-level (DL) matches from comprehension-level (CL) matches illustrates that researchers have really been asking two different questions. A study matching on comprehension is investigating whether the relative contributions of the subskills determining comprehension ability are the same in skilled and less skilled readers. Studies that match subjects purely on the basis of decoding ability are asking the same question within the more restricted domain of the word recognition module; that is, they are asking whether the two groups perform equally on word recognition tests for the same or different reasons.

Consider, for example, the implications for the predictions derived from the developmental lag hypothesis if the matching in an RL study is done with a comprehension test and dyslexics—identified by strict discrepancy criteria—are the poor reader group. The two groups will presumably be close in intelligence. Of course, similar intelligence test scores at different ages mean different things in terms of the raw score or absolute level of performance on a given test or index of ability. Thus, when older dyslexics are matched with younger children progressing normally in reading, the former will have higher raw scores on the intelligence measure. It should then also be the case that the dyslexics will score higher on any cognitive task that is correlated with the raw score on the intelligence test, and of course there are a host of such tasks. This has implications for the expected outcome in a CL design.

The argument goes as follows. The best candidates for the critical loci of reading disability (see Stanovich, 1986b, 1988) are tasks tapping a "vertical" faculty (i.e., processes operating in a specific domain; see Fodor, 1983) that is closely associated with reading but relatively dissociated from intelligence. According to the lag model, dyslexics lag in the development of certain vertical faculties and, as a result, their reading progress also lags. But consider that on any "horizontal" faculty, cognitive processes (those operating across a variety of domains) like metacognitive awareness, problem solving, and higher level language skills, the dyslexic should outperform the younger children (due to a higher mental age). However, then the reading test is a comprehension test, rather than a word recognition measure, the comprehension requirements of the test will implicate many of these higher level processes. Thus, the psychometric constraints imposed by the matching in a CL investigation should result in a pattern that I have previously characterized as compensatory processing (Stanovich, Nathan, & Vala-Rossi, 1986).

The compensatory processing hypothesis begins by assuming the importance of phonological processing skills in early reading development (Bradley & Bryant, 1985; Liberman, 1982; Mann, 1986; Stanovich, 1986b, 1988; Williams, 1984). From this assumption, and the psychometric constraints mentioned above, it follows that a rigorously defined sample of reading disabled children should display performance inferior to that of the younger CL-matched children on phonological analysis and phonological recoding skills, but should simultaneously display superior vocabulary, real-world knowledge, and/or strategic abilities (i.e., superior performance on other variables that should be correlated with the raw score on the IQ test). The similar overall level of comprehension ability in the two groups presumably obtains because the dyslexic children use these other skills and knowledge sources to compensate for seriously deficient phonological processing skills.

THE DEVELOPMENTAL LAG HYPOTHESIS AND THE GARDEN-VARIETY POOR READER

The situation is different when the lag hypothesis is applied to CL comparisons involving less skilled readers defined simply on the basis of reading ability relative to age. Such children are not statistically precluded from matching the complete cognitive performance profile of younger children who read at the same level. It is thus possible that population differences are the source of some of the empirical discrepancies in RL designs. These studies, like many in the dyslexia/LD literature, often fail to obtain a close IQ match between the dyslexic and nondisabled groups (Stanovich, 1986a; Torgesen & Dice, 1980). According to the hypotheses outlined here, any mismatch on IQ in a CL study will tend to change the pattern of results.

With respect to the specifically disabled reader, I have argued that the interrelations of the processes that determine comprehension are different from the two groups in a CL match. However, it is important to note that even if compensatory processing does explain the similar levels of comprehension, this does not necessarily guarantee the applicability of an analogous explanation of similar levels of decoding in a DL match. That is, it is perfectly possible that the comprehension ability of disabled readers is determined by compensatory processing (relative to younger CL controls), but that the operation of their word recognition modules is similar (in terms of regularity effects, orthographic processing, context effects, etc.) when compared to that of younger DL controls. (Note that from the compensatory hypothesis it follows that the DL match controls for an older disabled group of readers will not completely overlap with the disabled group's CL controls.)

Thus, in the case of the CL match, the finding of similar profiles across a wide variety of reading-related tasks is most likely to be observed with garden-variety poor readers. Such a finding would have implications for our understanding of specific reading disability, because it follows that when one of these groups (garden-variety vs. dyslexic poor readers) displays a profile match in a broad-based CL study, the other is logically precluded from doing so. In short, if we could nail down one of the possible data patterns in one of the populations of interest, the decreasing degrees of freedom would go a long way toward constraining further theoretical speculation. This, then, is the theoretical background that motivates the question we have asked in the research to be reported: Do garden-variety poor readers show matching profiles in a multivariate CL match that probes a variety of reading-related cognitive skills? I will report on two separate CL comparisons that are defined by a longitudinal research design.

A GARDEN-VARIETY CL MATCH

Our investigation began as a multivariate study of the reading-related cognitive subskills of third- and fifth-grade children. The far left column of Table 2.1 displays the variables in this investigation. The main criterion variable was the score on the Reading Survey Test of the Metropolitan Achievement Tests (Prescott, Balow, Hogan, & Farr, 1978), which is a test of reading comprehension. The Peabody Pic-

TABLE 2.1
Intercorrelations of All Variables

Variable	1	2	3	4	5	6	7	8	9	10	11	12	13	14
1. Metropolitan		.76*	-.50*	-.17	-.44*	-.02	-.07	-.18	-.16	-.45*	-.33*	-.72*	-.53*	.47*
2. PPVT[a]	.64*		-.48*	-.10	-.25	-.02	-.08	.00	.03	-.37*	-.15	-.51*	-.22	.59*
3. Rhyme Production Errors	-.43*	-.37*		.29*	.43*	.29*	.00	.12	-.25	.42*	.00	.50*	.35*	-.37*
4. Rhyme Production Time	-.29*	-.26	.24		.21	.06	-.20	-.14	.01	.28	.14	.20	.29*	.10
5. Oddity Errors	-.38*	-.36*	.42*	.33*		.36*	-.02	.25	-.04	.42*	.16	.50*	.45*	-.19
6. Oddity Time	-.29*	-.14	.30*	-.06	.13		.16	.15	.01	.22	.11	.26	.23	.11
7. Letter-Naming Time	-.30*	-.42*	.41*	.16	-.04	.16		.25	-.09	.02	-.06	.13	.00	-.25
8. Picture-Naming Time	-.38*	-.40*	.30*	.07	.18	.33*	.49*		-.15	-.16	-.20	.10	.00	-.20
9. Pseudoword-Naming Time	-.76*	-.54*	.67*	.30*	.30*	.31*	.43*	.48*		.23	.89*	.27	.33*	.06
10. Pseudoword-Naming Errors	-.52*	-.46*	.74*	.26	.42*	.18	.36*	.38*	.72*		.65*	.64*	.67*	-.08
11. Pseudoword z-Score	-.73*	-.55*	.73*	.31*	.36*	.29*	.43*	.48*	.97*	.86*		.51*	.57*	.01
12. Word Naming— Related Contexts	-.57*	-.36*	.34*	.15	.14	-.02	.27	.40*	.67*	.52*	.67*		.85*	-.45*
13. Word Naming— Neutral Contexts	-.71*	-.53*	.61*	.23	.31*	.28*	.46*	.48*	.91*	.67*	.89*	.80*		.08
14. Contextual Facilitation	-.36*	-.35*	.53*	.17	.30*	.48*	.37*	.22	.53*	.36*	.51*	-.11	.51*	

Correlations for the third-grade children are above the diagonal, and correlations for the fifth-grade children are below the diagonal.
[a]PPVT = Peabody Picture Vocabulary Test; *p < .05.

ture Vocabulary Test (Dunn, 1965) was employed as a measure of receptive vocabulary. Two measures of phonological sensitivity were employed: a rhyme production task and the odd-sound-out task popularized by Bradley and Bryant (1978, 1985). Response time, as well as errors, was assessed on these two tasks in an attempt to determine whether, for children of this age, speed might have a diagnosticity that accuracy lacks due to ceiling effects. In addition, it was thought that the speed instructions might serve to create more errors in the tasks and thus preclude ceiling effects that would ordinarily occur with children of this age.

Discrete-trial letter- and picture-naming tasks were included because previous investigators (e.g., Denckla & Rudel, 1976; Wolf, 1984) have linked deficiencies in naming speed and accuracy to reading problems. Pseudoword naming, an indicator of phonological recoding ability and potent predictor of reading ability at all levels, is associated with three variables in Table 2.1. Since both accuracy and speed have tended to be diagnostic, both were assessed. In addition, overall pseudoword naming skill was assessed by combining z-score indices for both time and accuracy into a composite z-score variable. Word naming was assessed under two conditions: with and without a related prior context (here termed the neutral and related conditions). These two conditions were administered using the contextual priming methodology that Richard West and I have utilized extensively (see Stanovich & West, 1983; West & Stanovich, 1978, 1982, 1986). A derived contextual facilitation variable was constructed by simply subtracting the mean time for word naming with related contexts from the mean time for word naming with neutral contexts.

Table 2.1 displays the intercorrelations among all of the variables for the third-grade children above the diagonal and for the fifth-grade children below the diagonal. Although there are many interesting relationships here, I will draw attention only to the top row where the correlations with the Metropolitan scores are displayed. The strongest predictors of reading comprehension are scores on the Peabody and word naming times (particularly in related contexts). The phonological sensitivity tasks and pseudoword naming errors are also moderate predictors. The far left column of correlations reveals similar, but not identical, relationships for the fifth-grade children. Here, every variable displayed a statistically significant relationship with reading ability, the strongest correlations involving pseudoword and word naming, in addition to the Peabody.

Table 2.2 presents the data of greatest interest. Here, the children in each grade are partitioned into skilled and less skilled readers, and the mean on each variable is presented for each group. Importantly, the partitioning was done so that the skilled third-grade children and

TABLE 2.2
Means for Each Task as a Function of Grade and Skill

Variable	Less Skilled Third Grade	Skilled Third Grade	Less Skilled Fifth Grade	Skilled Fifth Grade	Grade $F_{(1,60)}$	Skill $F_{(1,60)}$	Interaction $F_{(1,60)}$	Skilled Third Grade vs Less Skilled Fifth Grade $t_{(34)}$
PPVT[a]	64.8	78.0	78.6	92.4	38.68*	35.40*	0.02	-0.26
Rhyme Production Errors	2.93	1.06	1.33	0.43	9.62*	15.03*	1.83	-0.60
Rhyme Production Time	1117	1050	953	937	5.92*	0.51	0.20	1.39
Oddity Errors	6.71	4.61	4.89	3.71	4.49*	6.51*	0.52	-0.33
Oddity Time	693	584	563	482	3.67	2.50	0.05	0.27
Letter-Naming Time	581	576	518	497	25.96*	0.81	0.32	3.16*
Picture-Naming Time	829	756	771	702	3.70	5.97*	0.01	-0.39
Pseudoword-Naming Time	984	956	870	696	13.81*	4.03*	2.13	1.12
Pseudoword-Naming Errors	3.43	1.44	2.11	0.64	3.67	9.75*	0.22	-0.88
Pseudoword z-Score	0.64	0.12	-0.11	-1.14	13.42*	8.09*	0.87	0.55
Word Naming—Related Contexts	672	508	494	463	30.54*	23.15*	10.63*	0.59
Word Naming—Neutral Contexts	763	642	624	549	28.55*	20.08*	1.13	0.70
Contextual Facilitation	92	134	130	86	0.11	0.01	8.14*	0.26

[a]PPVT = Peabody Picture Vocabulary Test; *$p < .05$.

the less skilled fifth-grade children formed a comprehension-level match, both obtaining similar grade equivalent scores on the Metropolitan (5.2 and 5.1, respectively). The critical comparisons are thus represented in the second and third columns from the left. A statistical test of the means for each variable for the CL-matched groups is presented in the far right column.

The results of the CL comparisons are easily summarized. The performance patterns of these two groups were remarkably convergent. They differed significantly on only 1 of the 13 variables listed in Table 2.2. The performance of the two groups was virtually identical on the Peabody, rhyme-production errors, oddity errors, oddity response time, picture naming, pseudoword z-score, word naming speed in both related and neutral contexts, and contextual facilitation score. The fifth-grade children were 97 msec faster on the rhyme production task, but this difference was not significant. The fifth-grade students were also somewhat faster at pseudoword naming (again, not significantly so), but there are indications that this difference may be due to differential speed/accuracy tradeoff criteria. Although the fifth-grade readers were somewhat faster at pseudoword naming, they made more errors than the third-grade readers. Consistent with the idea of a conservative criterion among the skilled third graders was the finding that skill differences within this grade were large in the error rates (3.43 vs. 1.44) but small in the naming times (984 msec vs. 956 msec). Given a possible difference in speed/accuracy criteria in the two age groups, the best comparison of performance on pseudowords is the z-score variable, where both performance indices are combined. On this variable the two CL-matched groups were very similar.

Thus, only one variable—letter-naming time—differentiated the two groups. This variable has been shown to track age much more strongly than reading ability in previous investigations (Jackson & Biemiller, 1985; Stanovich, Feeman, & Cunningham, 1983), and so its statistical significance in a CL match is predictable and empirically convergent. With this one exception, the reading-related cognitive performance profiles of these two groups of readers were highly similar. This pattern of performance similarities is consistent with a developmental lag model of the reading skill deficits displayed by the less skilled fifth-grade children that extends over rather broad cognitive domains. Cognitively, they resemble younger children who are at the same stage of reading acquisition.

Two years later we conducted a similar investigation that had some new design features (Stanovich et al., 1988). First, we tested children in three grades—third, fifth, and seventh—and formed a three-group CL match spanning all three grades. Virtually all such designs in the current literature involve only two-group comparisons. Embedded within this new multivariate investigation was a longitudinal follow-up of the third- and fifth-grade children in the previous investigation, now fifth and seventh graders, respectively. These children, plus additional children not tested before, formed part of the larger sample in the second investigation. This second testing enabled us to examine a situation virtually unreported in the literature and one with some interesting theoretical implications: namely, a longitudinal comparison of groups of children who, 2 years earlier, had been CL matched.

The Metropolitan Reading Survey Test was again the criterion reading measure. The tasks that were carried over into the follow-up study were the Peabody, letter naming, rhyming, pseudoword naming, word recognition, and contextual facilitation. The oddity task and picture naming were eliminated. Replacing them were several new tasks and variables dictated by developments in reading research and theory. Motivated by Cohen's work (e.g., Cohen, 1982; Cohen & Netley, 1981; Cohen, Netley, & Clarke, 1984) showing differential linkages between various types of memory tasks and reading ability, we adapted two memory tasks—one relatively nonstrategic and the other intended to be strategy loaded—for use in a multivariate battery like this one. The nonstrategic task was an adaptation of the running serial memory task investigated by Cohen and Netley (1981). The speed and unpredictability of the end of the stimulus sequence serve to preclude the use of memory strategies in the task. The strategic memory task was an adaptation of Brown's (1972) "keeping track" task, judged to be relatively strategy loaded.

In this investigation the words named under neutral contextual conditions were subdivided in order to allow us to examine another variable. Half of the stimuli were regular words having common spelling-to-sound correspondences, and half were exception words having uncommon spelling-to-sound correspondences (stimuli were chosen from those used in the investigation of Treiman & Hirsh-Pasek, 1985). Some recent studies (e.g., Backman, Bruck, Hebert, & Seidenberg, 1984; Manis, 1985; Morrison, 1984, 1987; Waters, Seidenberg, & Bruck, 1984) have indicated that more skilled readers may display smaller spelling-to-sound regularity effects, presumably because of greater reliance on visual/orthographic mechanisms to mediate lexical access. Several theorists have viewed regularity effects as a window on the mechanisms operating in the word recognition module. Thus, regularity effects are the type of indicator one wants when comparing children of different ages who have arrived at similar levels of reading ability.

A final new measure was an articulation speed task adapted from the work of Hulme, Thomson, Muir, and Lawrence (1984). These investigators have linked articulation speed to memory span, and Manis (1985) has observed a difference of 50 msec in production latency (the time to initiate the pronunciation of a known word) between disabled and nondisabled readers. Theoretically, the recent emphasis on the critical importance of the operation of the phonological module in the development of individual differences in reading (Liberman & Shankweiler, 1985; Mann, 1986; Stanovich, 1986b) also motivates an interest in articulation speed. While no theorist believes that the critical differences are actually located at the articulatory level, it could be that articulation speed taps into the module in a way that would make it act as a marker variable for phonological problems at deeper levels (see also Catts, 1986).

Table 2.3 contains a listing of all the variables that were analyzed, along with the means for each of six groups defined by the factorial combination of grade and skill level based on a median split within each grade. Clearly, the comparisons of skill within each grade resulted in many significant differences. Perhaps a more comprehensible presentation of the results is contained in Tables 2.4 and 2.5, which display correlation matrices for a selected set of the variables. In order to reduce the size of these matrices, composite z-score variables were used for the rhyming task, pseudoword naming, regularity effect, and word naming in neutral context. Focusing again on the predictors of performance on the Metropolitan, we see that for the third-grade children (above the diagonal in Table 2.4), the strongest relationships were with pseudoword and word naming and to a lesser extent with the Peabody. For the fifth-grade children (below the diagonal, column one), the best predictors were word naming and the Peabody. For the seventh graders (Table 2.5), the Peabody was the best predictor, followed by pseudoword and word naming.

More important are the results displayed in Table 2.6, which are the means for the three CL-matched groups. It should be noted that because the fifth- and seventh-grade children took the same test, the match for these two groups was particularly good since they could be equated on actual raw scores. The third-grade children, who completed the Elementary rather than the Intermediate form of the test, were matched on grade equivalents and thus their match is psychometrically less secure. The resulting three groups represented a seventh-grade group considerably below average for their age, a fifth-grade group that is below average, and a third-grade group of above-average ability.

Table 2.6 indicates that only two of the variables differed significantly across the three CL-matched groups. Letter naming was significantly faster for older children. This variable, however, was unrelated to reading ability (see Table 2.3). Thus, this study replicated the finding in our previous study and in the work of other investigators (e.g., Jackson & Biemiller, 1985) that letter-naming speed tracks chronological age more strongly than reading ability. The other variable

TABLE 2.3
Means of Variables for Skilled and Less Skilled Readers in Each Grade

Variable	Third Grade			Fifth Grade			Seventh Grade		
	Skilled	Less Skilled	$t(38)$	Skilled	Less Skilled	$t(40)$	Skilled	Less Skilled	$t(42)$
Metropolitan raw score	45.4	23.8	10.31**	48.2	28.1	11.55**	52.0	32.1	10.46**
Metropolitan grade equivalent	4.35	2.37	5.64**	8.00	4.02	9.07	9.73	4.60	8.42**
PPVT[a]	73.4	69.8	1.45	83.4	73.9	3.25	91.7	76.5	4.67**
Strategic memory task	14.1	12.5	1.86	15.0	14.1	1.21	16.0	14.8	1.71
Nonstrategic memory task (items)	27.3	23.4	2.23*	28.6	26.8	1.18	30.0	28.9	.78
Nonstrategic memory task (order)	21.3	15.2	2.66*	20.4	18.4	1.11	23.0	20.3	1.37
Letter-naming time	533	575	1.81	505	500	.26	461	474	1.04
Regular word-naming time	666	892	3.00**	633	648	.45	557	678	2.68*
Regular word-naming errors	1.30	2.60	3.19**	.76	1.81	3.53**	1.05	1.64	2.06*
Exception word-naming time	706	1006	4.27**	648	679	.99	588	743	3.12**
Exception word-naming errors	2.20	4.15	3.97**	1.05	2.00	3.13**	1.32	2.00	1.88
Mean neutral word-naming time	686	949	3.73**	641	663	.80	573	711	3.12**
Mean neutral word-naming errors	1.75	3.38	4.10**	.90	1.90	3.94**	1.18	1.82	2.40
Neutral word z-score	-.061	1.260	4.42**	-.514	-.056	3.77**	-.577	.030	3.62**
Regularity effect (times)	40	114	2.04*	15	31	.58	32	65	.96
Regularity effect (errors)	.90	1.55	1.51	.29	.19	.30	.27	.36	.24
Regularity z-score	.084	.671	2.49*	-.269	-.232	.21	-.197	-.011	.86
Related word-naming time	518	675	2.89**	482	485	.16	422	495	3.77**
Related word-naming errors	.35	1.50	2.81**	.05	.48	3.07**	.14	.14	.00
Contextual facilitation	168	274	2.19*	159	178	.80	151	216	1.95
Pseudoword-naming time	828	1304	4.24**	807	854	.69	652	952	4.11**
Pseudoword-naming errors	2.75	7.25	5.55**	1.86	2.71	1.34	1.14	3.95	3.83**
Pseudoword z-score	-.181	1.267	5.84**	-.358	-.147	1.31	-.707	.202	4.48**
Rhyming reaction time	1098	1127	.38	924	1058	1.74	1056	1081	.36
Rhyming errors	4.05	4.08	1.06	2.57	4.19	2.42*	2.68	4.14	2.42*
Rhyming z-score	.157	.348	.82	-.527	.107	2.44*	-.232	.142	1.60
Articulation time	9290	9447	.37	8334	8577	.73	7604	7298	1.34

*Difference between skilled and less skilled readers significant at the .05 level (two-tailed test).
**Difference between skilled and less skilled readers significant at the .01 level (two-tailed test).
[a]PPVT = Peabody Picture Vocabulary Test.

TABLE 2.4
Intercorrelations of Variables for Third- and Fifth-Grade Children

Variable	1	2	3	4	5	6	7	8	9	10	11
1. Metropolitan		.50	.29	.29	-.13	-.34	-.21	-.69	-.38	-.37	-.72
2. PPVT[a]	.51		.22	.05	-.44	-.25	-.01	-.24	-.15	-.01	-.28
3. Strategic Memory Task	.15	.19		.28	-.13	-.30	-.15	-.12	-.20	-.15	-.15
4. Nonstrategic Memory Task (correct order)	.25	.26	.05		-.05	-.23	-.25	-.03	-.08	.01	-.27
5. Articulation Time	-.03	.04	.05	-.23		.46	-.08	.00	-.08	.24	.20
6. Letter-Naming Time	.02	.06	.08	.02	.54		.44	.36	.28	.30	.49
7. Rhyming z-Score	-.32	-.03	-.17	-.16	.37	.17		.42	.21	.22	.41
8. Neutral Word z-Score	-.56	-.18	-.01	-.22	.19	.03	.39		.26	.56	.69
9. Regularity z-Score	-.03	-.15	-.03	.03	-.17	-.06	-.02	-.06		-.09	.35
10. Contextual Facilitation	-.19	-.08	.00	-.17	.07	.08	-.12	.42	-.09		.46
11. Pseudoword z-Score	-.22	-.13	.00	-.13	.04	.07	.14	.36	-.10	.46	

Correlations for the third-grade children are above the diagonal, and correlations for the fifth-grade children are below the diagonal.
Correlations above .31 are significant at the .05 level (two-tailed).
[a]PPVT = Peabody Picture Vocabulary Test.

TABLE 2.5
Intercorrelations of Variables for Seventh-Grade Children

Variable	1	2	3	4	5	6	7	8	9	10	11
1. Metropolitan		.70	.31	.31	.05	-.36	-.34	-.59	-.20	-.37	-.62
2. PPVT[a]			.30	.18	-.05	-.18	-.19	-.43	-.06	-.22	-.55
3. Strategic Memory Task				.23	.04	-.10	-.12	-.29	-.17	-.23	-.42
4. Nonstrategic Memory Task (correct order)					.02	-.19	-.30	-.43	-.10	-.43	-.47
5. Articulation Time						.50	.06	-.09	-.04	.13	-.02
6. Letter-Naming Time							.05	.43	.05	.44	.36
7. Rhyming z-Score								.27	.08	.25	.25
8. Neutral Word z-Score									.31	.70	.77
9. Regularity z-Score										.08	.15
10. Contextual Facilitation											.76
11. Pseudoword z-Score											

Correlations above .29 are significant at the .05 level (two-tailed).
[a]PPVT = Peabody Picture Vocabulary Test.

TABLE 2.6
Means for Groups Matched on Reading Ability

Variable	Third Grade	Fifth Grade	Seventh Grade	F(2,61)
Metropolitan grade equivalent	4.35	4.32	4.37	.01
PPVT[a]	73.4	74.4	76.7	.97
Strategic memory task	14.1	14.3	14.6	.24
Nonstrategic memory task (items)	27.3	26.8	28.5	.57
Nonstrategic memory task (order)	21.3	18.2	19.6	1.35
Letter-naming time	533	503	477	4.37*
Regular word-naming time	666	652	695	.50
Regular word-naming errors	1.30	1.64	1.58	.60
Exception word-naming time	706	678	752	1.23
Exception word-naming errors	2.20	1.88	2.05	.42
Mean neutral word-naming time	686	665	723	.98
Mean neutral word-naming errors	1.75	1.76	1.82	.03
Neutral word z-score	−.061	−.109	.061	.58
Regularity effect (times)	42	25	57	.45
Regularity effect (errors)	.90	.24	.47	1.93
Regularity z-score	.084	−.239	−.005	1.51
Related word-naming time	518	487	498	1.15
Related word-naming errors	.35	.40	.16	1.36
Contextual facilitation	168	178	226	1.56
Pseudoword-naming time	828	841	937	.89
Pseudoword-naming errors	2.75	2.48	4.05	2.07
Pseudoword z-score	−.181	−.205	.196	2.06
Rhyming reaction time	1098	999	1094	1.12
Rhyming errors	4.05	3.88	4.47	.47
Rhyming z-score	.157	−.082	.243	.91
Articulation time	9290	8471	7298	17.76**

[a]PPVT = Peabody Picture Vocabulary Test, *$p < .05$; **$p < .001$.

to show a significant difference—articulation time—displayed a pattern similar to letter-naming time, although in even stronger form. As is clear from Tables 2.3 through 2.5, articulation time appears to be completely unrelated to reading ability. However, it is strongly related to chronological age. Overall, then, with the exception of two variables that are relatively unrelated to reading ability, the performance profiles of these three groups of children displayed remarkable similarity. They had similar vocabularies, strategic and nonstrategic memory abilities, and rhyming ability. Their word recognition processes were very similar, as indicated by their context effects, regularity effects, and pseudoword naming ability.

There are several reasons why this uniformity of performance among the three CL-matched groups is striking. First, it is noteworthy in light of the varied set of tasks employed. Most previous RL-match investigations have used a much more restricted battery of tasks. In addition, when such a large number of statistical tests are run on a set of variables, some spurious significant differences could well appear. Also, one might worry if nonsignificant statistical results were observed in the presence of large absolute differences between the means, which might indicate that large variability and/or small sample sizes were rendering real differences nondetectable. However, this was clearly not the case, as in most instances the mean performance levels of the three groups were quite close (the possible exception being pseudoword naming). Finally, the analyses on the median splits (see Table 2.3) indicate that the design and measurement techniques were powerful enough to detect differences.

THE LONGITUDINAL COMPARISON

As mentioned previously, subgroups of the fifth- and seventh-grade children tested in 1986 had been tested 2 years earlier (in 1984), as third and fifth graders, respectively. Individual differences in reading achievement were quite stable. Correlations between Metropolitan raw scores in 1984 and 1986 were .93 and .78 for the fifth- and seventh-grade children, respectively. Table 2.7 presents the correlations between the 1986 Metropolitan scores and the variables assessed 2 years earlier. In general, the variables that predicted 1986 achievement were the same variables that had predicted concurrent achievement in 1984. More interesting is the longitudinal comparison involving the previously CL-matched groups. What does the performance of these two groups—which 2 years earlier had been as displayed in Table 2.2—look like 2 years later? Are they still a CL match? The performance of these two groups—matched on reading comprehension performance in 1984—is compared on the variables administered 2 years later in Table 2.8. Interestingly, the two groups are now no longer matched on reading comprehension ability. The raw scores on the Metropolitan Reading Survey are significantly different. In terms of grade equivalents, the skilled younger readers showed a gain of 2.8 years during the 2-year period compared with 1.5 for the older less skilled readers. The results from the other variables do not indicate a large number of differences. However, there were significant tendencies for the younger readers to be superior in word-naming accuracy in neutral contexts and in rhyme performance. The older children were sig-

TABLE 2.7
Correlations Between Reading Ability and Tasks Administered 2 Years Earlier

Variable	Fifth-Grade Children	Seventh-Grade Children
PPVT[a]	.74	.58
Rhyming errors	−.47	−.42
Rhyming time	−.15	−.26
Phonological oddity errors	−.53	−.49
Phonological oddity time	−.15	−.21
Letter-naming time	−.04	−.31
Picture-naming time	−.30	−.38
Pseudoword-naming time	−.12	−.61
Pseudoword-naming errors	−.23	−.59
Pseudoword z-score	−.24	−.65
Related word-naming time	−.53	−.34
Neutral word-naming time	−.38	−.51
Contextual facilitation	.44	−.37

Correlations above .40 and .38 are significant at the .05 level (two-tailed) for the fifth- and seventh-grade children, respectively.
[a]PPVT = Peabody Picture Vocabulary Test.

nificantly faster in the articulation task, a finding anticipated by the previous results indicating that this task is strongly linked to chronological age.

Most versions of the developmental lag hypothesis posit that there are acquisition rate differences between readers of differing skill: that skilled and less skilled readers go through the same sequence of stages but at different rates. The hypothesis of rate differences clearly predicts that the younger skilled readers should show more growth in reading in a fixed amount of time than the older less skilled readers. Most of the previous and conflicting research on this issue (e.g., Baker, Decker, & DeFries, 1984; Bruck, 1988; Trites & Fiedorowicz, 1976) has compared groups of similar chronological age but differing initial reading levels. Thus, the hypothesis must be assessed by evaluating a group by time interaction that is vulnerable to many artifacts. Perhaps a longitudinal CL-match design provides a less artifact-ridden method of assessing whether there are differential growth rates. Our results appear to reveal the predicted differential reading growth rates.

In summary, the results from the three-group CL-match longitudinal design converged with our earlier results. Both sets of results confirmed the hypothesis (Stanovich et al., 1986a, 1986b) that the performance of unlabeled poor readers—those children who read poorly but do not necessarily fit the psychometric criteria for the label

TABLE 2.8
Performance of Groups Matched on Reading Ability in 1984
on the Tasks Administered in 1986

Variable	Skilled Fifth-Grade Children	Less Skilled Seventh-Grade Children	t(26)
Metropolitan raw score	48.1	39.5	2.38*
Metropolitan grade equivalent	7.94	6.59	1.38
PPVT[a]	85.7	84.4	.36
Strategic memory task	15.1	15.6	.91
Nonstrategic memory task (items)	29.6	29.4	.13
Nonstrategic memory task (order)	21.9	20.3	.81
Letter-naming time	489	470	.99
Regular word-naming time	604	623	.41
Regular word-naming errors	.36	1.43	5.61**
Exception word-naming time	625	640	.34
Exception word-naming errors	.93	2.14	3.61**
Mean neutral word-naming time	614	632	.38**
Mean neutral word-naming errors	.64	1.79	5.43**
Neutral word z-score	−.687	−.184	3.74**
Regularity effect (times)	21	17	.20
Regularity effect (errors)	.57	.71	.41
Regularity z-score	−.133	−.096	.23
Related word-naming time	469	448	.73
Related word-naming errors	.07	.21	1.06
Contextual facilitation	145	184	.98
Pseudoword-naming time	789	746	.53
Pseudoword-naming errors	2.00	2.36	.33
Pseudoword z-score	−.362	−.367	.02
Rhyming reaction time	984	1140	1.93
Rhyming errors	2.36	3.50	1.76
Rhyming z-score	−.453	.121	2.18*
Articulation time	8131	7266	2.34*

[a]PPVT = Peabody Picture Vocabulary Test; *$p<.05$; **$p<.01$.

dyslexia—would show a broad-based developmental lag. It is hypothesized that this pattern will contrast with the results from studies where the reading-level match involves reading disabled children defined by strict psychometric criteria.

A RESEARCH SYNTHESIS

In the following discussion I will try to amalgamate a number of findings and theoretical ideas into a coherent global model for understanding reading problems of both the garden-variety and dyslexic type. Although the "grain" of the model will be rather coarse, I would argue that we are better off with even a gross summary if it can help us to escape from the interminable definitional and semantic disputes that plague the LD field—and I think that my model does do this. My summary model builds on the basic result regarding garden-variety readers that I feel my work has established. It supplements this empirical finding with some of the logical, statistical, and psychometric arguments that began my chapter. Not the least important, however, is my reliance on the previous theoretical arguments and empirical results established by other investigators.

Here is what I think has been roughly established. First, Andrew Ellis (1985) is right that the proper analogy for dyslexia is not measles, but instead a condition like obesity. There is considerable evidence from a variety of different sources (Jorm, 1983; Olson et al., 1985; Scarborough, 1984; Seidenberg et al., 1985; Share, McGee, McKenzie, Williams, & Silva, 1987; Silva et al., 1985) that we are not dealing with a discrete entity but with a graded continuum. Several years ago, Rutter and Yule (1975) led researchers down a blind alley by reporting that there was a somewhat discontinuous "hump" near the bottom of the reading distribution, and this hump suggested a discrete pathology model to many investigators. However, there is now much converging evidence that indicates that the hump was a statistical artifact, perhaps involving ceiling effects on the tests (Rodgers, 1983; Share et al., 1987; Silva et al., 1985; Van der Wissel & Zegers, 1985). There is in fact no hump in the distribution.

However, the fact that the distribution is a graded continuum does not render the concept of dyslexia scientifically useless, as many critics would like to argue. This is why obesity is such a good example—no one doubts that it is a real health problem, despite the fact that it is operationally defined in a somewhat arbitrary way by choosing a criterion in a continuous distribution:

> For people of any given age and height there will be an uninterrupted continuum from painfully thin to inordinately fat. It is entirely arbitrary where we draw the line between "normal" and "obese," but that does not prevent obesity being a real and worrying condition, nor does it prevent research into the causes and cures of obesity being both valuable and necessary. (Ellis, 1985, p. 172)

It follows that, "To ask how prevalent dyslexia is in the general population will be as meaningful, and as meaningless, as asking how prevalent obesity is. The answer will depend entirely upon where the line is drawn" (p. 172).

Likewise, I think that it is also important to conceive of *all* of the relevant distributions of reading-related cognitive skills as being continuously arrayed in a multidimensional space and not distributed in clusters. In short, I accept the model of heterogeneity without clustering that has been discussed by Ellis (1985), Olson et al. (1985), Satz, Morris, and Fletcher (1985), and others. I further posit that the existence of heterogeneity without clustering is precisely the empirical fact that has obscured and stymied the search for discrete subtypes among dyslexic children. Ellis (1985) illustrates the idea with a figure that I think is instructive (see Figure 2.1). It doesn't tell us anything new, but it does shift our thinking into a quantitative mode, which often helps to clarify precisely the things that the verbal debate obscures because of the inherent connotations of discreteness carried by many natural language terms.

In Figure 2.1, the categorical model implicit in many discussions of dyslexic subtypes is illustrated on the left. This is the model that motivated the earlier, more naive attempts at finding a dyslexia typology. The two dimensions (note that all of the same arguments would apply in a space of higher dimension) represent ability at accessing the lexicon on a visual/orthographic basis (termed "whole word reading" on Ellis's X-axis) and phonological recoding ability (termed "phonic reading" on Ellis's Y-axis). The categorical model assumes that there are "galaxies" of dyslexics—and of nondyslexic readers as well. If this model were true, the subtyping literature would not have remained so confused for so long. Nevertheless, it is worthwhile to consider the figure further. In it, we can identify the dysphonetic and dyseidetic dyslexic typology popularized by Boder (1973) and somewhat recapitulated in the distinction between phonological and surface dyslexia in the literature on acquired dyslexia. These two groups are defined by severe deficits on one of the dimensions and normal ability on the other. Since both abilities are necessary for fluent reading, the result of both of these patterns is a disabled reader. In the lower left are the unfortunate individuals handicapped by deficits in both word recognition mechanisms. The other two clusters are two subtypes of fluent readers, the so-called Chinese and Phoenicians—extremely facile at one type of lexical access mechanism, but with normal skill on the other (see Baron & Strawson, 1976; Treiman & Baron, 1984).

The right side of Figure 2.1 portrays what Ellis calls the "dimensional model." The poor readers in the lower left quadrant are a heterogeneous lot, but they do not form clusters. Like Ellis and several other investigators (e.g., Olson et al., 1985), I believe that if we really want to have a useful concept of dyslexia, this is the model we must always keep in mind. Again, like in the obesity example, we may decide to arbitrarily cut the variability in the lower left and for various pur-

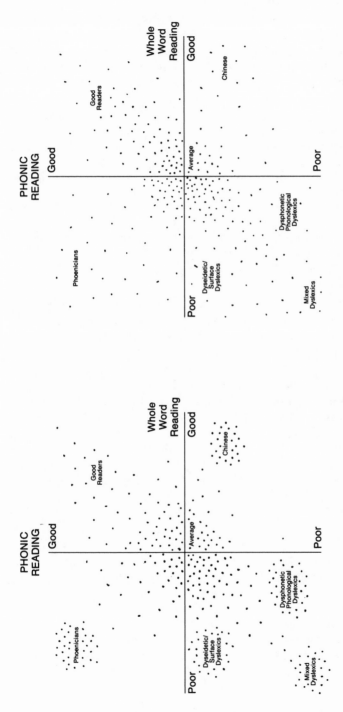

Figure 2.1. On the left side of the figure, hypothetical distribution on whole-word (direct-visual) reading skill and phonic (assembled, sublexical) reading skill of a sample of readers age 15 years or over with IQ = 100 +, on a categorical model. On the right side of the figure, hypothetical distribution of the same sample of readers but on a dimensional model. *Note.* From "The Cognitive Neuropsychology of Developmental (and Acquired) Dyslexia: A Critical Survey," 1985, *Cognitive Psychology, 2*(2), pp. 192, 193. Copyright 1985 by Lawrence Erlbaum Associates. Reprinted by permission.

poses treat the subgroups in a discrete fashion—but this again would be an arbitrarily imposed partitioning. Clearly, this state of affairs creates statistical problems for cluster analyses, but it is important to understand—via a logic similar to that in the obesity example—that such problems do not undermine the idea of forming abstract subtypes for certain theoretical or practical purposes:

> What the dimensional model predicts, however, is that there will be a complete and unbroken gradation of intermediate dyslexics linking such extreme cases. A dimensional model does not deny heterogeneity, only homogeneity of subtypes (cf. Olson, Kliegl, Davidson, & Foltz, 1985). It does not exclude the study of selected individuals to highlight dimensions of difference, nor does it prevent one from drawing conclusions about reading processes in general from the observed individual differences. It may, however, undermine an attempt to impose syndromes upon the dyslexic population. That is, the dimensional approach primarily creates problems for a syndrome-based version of preformism; other versions may be less affected by the denial of homogeneous subgroups. (Ellis, 1985, pp. 192–193)

Finally, it is important to notice that there is a great degree of heterogeneity within the normal sample as well (simply draw a line connecting the Phoenicians to the Chinese). This figure illustrates graphically why Bryant and Impey (1986) were able to find RL-matched younger children who showed the same extreme patterns as some of the well-known case studies of phonological and surface dyslexia. One can see, for example, how some Phoenicians who are adequate readers will display performance patterns as extreme as surface dyslexics on some tasks.

I would, however, modify Ellis's figure in one extremely important way. His scatter plot displays dysphonetics as roughly equal in frequency to dyseidetics. There is now voluminous data—some in Boder's (1973) classic paper itself—indicating that the dysphonetic pattern is far more common than the dyseidetic (Gough & Hillinger, 1980; Liberman, 1982; Liberman & Shankweiler, 1985; Pennington, 1986; Perfetti, 1985; Stanovich, 1986b, 1988; Vellutino, 1979). This fact meshes nicely with an interesting finding of Bryant and Impey (1986). There was only one performance pattern that they could not recapitulate with an RL-matched younger child: the extremely poor nonword reading of a phonological dyslexic (see Snowling et al., 1986). A greater bunching of phonological dyslexics at the bottom of the figure would make it more likely that certain outliers in this group would not find matches on phonological skills with nondyslexic readers in the lower right quadrant.

THE PHONOLOGICAL-CORE
VARIABLE-DIFFERENCE MODEL

The concepts inherent in the dimensional model outlined above can be generalized to account for contrasts between the dyslexic and the garden-variety poor reader. The bivariate distrubtion of reading and IQ is continuous, as is the univariate distribution of reading ability. What this means is that there is a continuous gradation between these two types of poor reader, defined by where they are on the bivariate relation of IQ and reading. That is, conditionalized at a given level of reading ability (low, in the case of the poor reader), the distribution of IQ is continuous, with an "unbroken gradation of intermediate cases" between the "pure" dyslexic (with relatively high IQ for that level of reading) and the "pure" garden-variety (with a lower and more typical IQ). This means that to whatever extent the processing patterns of these two groups are dissimilar, that dissimilarity will be attenuated the closer we get to the "fuzzy" and arbitrary boundary between them. Or, to put it more concretely, studies employing dyslexics with somewhat depressed IQs and garden-variety poor readers with somewhat elevated IQs may be unable to detect whatever critical processing differences there are between the two groups.

And I do believe that such processing differences exist. They can be described within what I will term the phonological-core variable-difference model; actually, perhaps more of a framework than a model. The model rests on a clear understanding of the assumption of specificity in definitions of dyslexia (see Hall & Humphreys, 1982; Stanovich, 1986a, 1986b). This assumption underlies all discussions of the concept of dyslexia, even if it is not explicitly stated. It is the idea that a child with this type of learning disability has a brain/cognitive deficit that is reasonably specific to the reading task. That is, the concept of dyslexia requires that the deficits displayed by such children not extend too far into other domains of cognitive functioning. If they did, this would depress the constellation of abilities we call intelligence, reduce the reading/intelligence discrepancy, and the child would no longer be dyslexic! Indeed, he or she would have become a garden variety!

In short, the key deficit in dyslexia must be a vertical faculty rather than a horizontal faculty (see Fodor, 1983); that is, a domain-specific process (Cossu & Marshall, 1986) rather than a process that operates across a wide variety of domains. For this and other reasons, many investigators have located the proximal locus of dyslexia at the word recognition level (e.g., Gough & Tunmer, 1986; Morrison, 1984, 1987; Perfetti, 1985; Siegel, 1985; Vellutino, 1979) and have been searching for the locus of the flaw in the word recognition module. Research in the last 10 years has focused intensively on phonological process-ing abilities. It is now well established that dyslexic children display deficits in various aspects of phonological processing. They have dif-ficulty making explicit reports about sound segments at the phoneme level, they display naming difficulties, they utilize phonological codes in short-term memory inefficiently, and they may have other-than-normal categorical perception of certain phonemes (see Liberman & Shankweiler, 1985; Mann, 1986; Pennington, 1986; Wagner & Torgesen, 1987; Williams, 1984). Importantly, there is increasing evidence that the linkage from phonological processing ability to reading skill is a causal one (Bradley & Bryant, 1985; Liberman & Shankweiler, 1985; Maclean, Bryant, & Bradley, 1987; Stanovich, 1986b, 1988; Wagner & Torgesen, 1987). Presumably, their lack of phonological sensitivity makes the learning of grapheme-to-phoneme correspondences very difficult.

The model of individual differences I will present thus posits this core of phonological deficits as the basis of the dyslexic performance pattern. This is an oversimplification, since it ignores—at least tem-porarily—the existence of those (admittedly many fewer) cases in the upper left corner of the poor reader quadrant in Figure 2.1: the dyseidetics, or surface dyslexics. I believe that there is growing evidence for the utility of distinguishing a group of dyslexics who have severe problems in accessing the lexicon on a visual/orthographic basis (see Stanovich, 1988). But a crucial caveat is in order. I believe that the problem encountered by these children is not similar to the "visual perception" problems popular in the early history of the study of dys-lexia, but now thoroughly debunked (Aman & Singh, 1983; Kavale & Mattson, 1983; Vellutino, 1979). In addition to the empirical evidence refuting this old view, the arguments presented here add to the negative convergence. The older conceptualizations of visual deficits had the additional flaw that the purported problematic processes were too global and not modular enough. The actual problems in orthographic processing must be much more subtle and localized. I am not prepared to say anything more specific about this issue, except that I would speculate that the problem involves the automatic and nonintentional induction of orthographic patterns (and thus would not be discerni-ble under most intentional learning situations, for example, most stan-dard paired-associate learning paradigms). However, the small group of dyslexics with orthographic-core deficits would mirror the phonological-core group in all of the other processing characteristics of the model. What are those characteristics?

One important factor mentioned earlier was that of compensatory processing. CL-matched younger children should display superior word recognition skill and phonological abilities, whereas the older dyslexics should display superior vocabulary, memory, and real-world knowledge—the latter skills and knowledge presumably balancing the inferior word recognition skills to yield the equivalent reading comprehension performance (see Bruck, 1988). A similar trade-off should characterize comparisons of dyslexics and garden-variety poor readers matched on comprehension: poorer word recognition but superior "horizontal faculties" on the part of the dyslexics. There is some evidence supportive of this trend (Bloom et al., 1980; Fredman & Stevenson, 1988; Seidenberg et al., 1985).

A DL match should yield complementary results. The older dyslexics, matched at the word recognition level, should display superior reading comprehension. Similarly, dyslexics matched with garden-variety chronological age (CA) controls on decoding skill should display superior reading comprehension and horizontal faculties (see Bloom et al., 1980; Ellis & Large, 1987; Jorm et al., 1986; Silva et al., 1985).

For the majority of dyslexics with a phonological-core deficit, a DL match with a younger group of nondyslexic controls should reveal another pattern of ability trade-offs: deficits in phonological sensitivity and in the phonological mechanisms that mediate lexical access—but superior visual/orthographic mechanisms and orthographic knowledge (an opposite but analogous pattern should obtain for those with an orthographic-core deficit). Several investigations have shown this predicted pattern (Baddeley et al., 1982; Baron & Treiman, 1980; Bradley & Bryant, 1978; Kochnower et al., 1983; Olson et al., 1985; Snowling, 1980, 1981). A similar pattern should hold when dyslexics are compared to a CA garden-variety group. These, then, are the patterns of relationships that can be derived from the phonological-core deficit of the dyslexic reader and the psychometric constraints inherent in the operational definition of dyslexia. (Note that Olson et al., 1985, have used similar ideas of compensatory processing to explain the variability *within* a dyslexic sample.)

In the phonological-core variable-difference model, the term *variable differences* is used to contrast the performance of the garden-variety and the dyslexic reader. As outlined above, the cognitive status of garden-variety poor readers is well described by a developmental lag model. Cognitively, they are remarkably similar to younger children reading at the same level. A logical corollary of this pattern is that the garden-variety reader will have a wide variety of cognitive deficits when compared to CA controls who are reading at normal levels.

However, it is important to understand that the garden-variety poor reader does share the phonological problems of the dyslexic reader—though perhaps in less severe form—and the deficits appear also to be a causal factor in the poor reading of these children (Perfetti,

1985; Stanovich, 1986b). But for them the deficits—relative to CA controls—extend into a variety of domains (see Ellis & Large, 1987), and some of these (e.g., vocabulary, language comprehension) may also be causally linked to reading comprehension. Such a pattern does not characterize the dyslexic, who has a deficit localized in the phonological core. This core deficit is actually more severe (they show deficits in DL matches) than that of the garden-variety reader—whose performance matches younger DL controls—but it is not accompanied by other cognitive limitations.

One straightforward prediction that we then might derive is that the dyslexic's decoding problem will be more difficult to remediate. Interestingly, however, if the decoding problem can be remediated, then the contingent prognosis for dyslexic children should be better—they have no additional cognitive problems that may inhibit reading comprehension growth. This prediction fits nicely with Gough and Tunmer's (1986) "simple view" of reading comprehension (R) as a multiplicative combination of decoding skill (D) and listening comprehension ability (C); in short, $R = D \times C$. If dyslexics and garden-variety poor readers are matched on reading comprehension (for example, $.4 \times .9 = .6 \times .6$) and if (in some benign world) we were to totally remediate the decoding deficits of each, then the dyslexics would have superior reading comprehension ($1.0 \times .9 > 1.0 \times .6$).

The framework of the phonological-core variable-difference model fits nicely with Ellis's dimensional model described earlier. Consider the following characterization: As we move in the multidimensional space—through the "unbroken gradation of intermediate cases"—from the dyslexic to the garden-variety poor reader, we will move from a processing deficit localized in the phonological core to the global deficits of the developmentally lagging garden-variety poor reader. Thus, the actual cognitive differences that are displayed will be variable depending upon the type of poor reader who is the focus of the investigation. The differences on one end of the continuum will consist of deficits located only in the phonological core (the dyslexic) and will increase in number as we run through the intermediate cases that are less and less likely to pass strict psychometric criteria for dyslexia. Eventually we will reach the part of the multidimensional space containing relatively "pure" garden-variety poor readers who clearly will not qualify for the label dyslexic (by either regression or exclusionary criteria), will have a host of cognitive deficits, and will have the cognitively immature profile of a developmentally lagging individual. As we travel in this direction through the space the phonological-core deficit will attenuate somewhat. That is, the phonological problem will attenuate in severity as the number of other deficits spreads. One would need an impressive multidimensional graphic to illustrate this more concretely, but I hope that the previous consideration of Ellis's figure has primed our imaginations.

I believe that this phonological-core variable-deficit (PCVD) conceptualization provides a useful global framework within which to consider the plethora of controversial issues in the area of reading disabilities—issues of definition, subtypes, prevalence, etiology, process analysis, educational policy, remediation, and prognosis. For example, the framework provides an explanation for why almost all processing investigations of reading disability have uncovered phonological deficits, but also why some investigations have found deficits in *other* areas as well. This outcome is predictable from the fact that the PCVD model posits that *all* poor readers have a phonological deficit, but that other processing deficits emerge as one drifts in the multidimensional space from "pure" dyslexics toward garden-variety poor readers. Thus, the model's straightforward prediction is that those studies that revealed a more isolated deficit will be those that had more psychometrically select dyslexic readers. In short, the reading/IQ discrepancy of the subject populations should be significantly greater in those studies displaying more specific deficits. Presumably, studies finding deficits extending beyond the phonological domain are in the "fuzzy" area of the multidimensional space and are picking up the increasing number of processing differences that extend beyond the phonological domain as one moves toward the garden-variety area of the space.

This example of how the PCVD model clarifies and explains problematic findings in the LD literature is not a trivial one. I have previously discussed (see Stanovich, 1986a) how the research findings indicating multiple and somewhat global deficits threaten to make nonsense of the very concept of a learning disability. Escaping this paradox is a not inconsiderable problem for the LD field.

Nevertheless, I should not imply that the further necessary elaboration and quantification of the model will be an easy task. Numerous complications threaten to obscure its basically simple structure. I have already mentioned the likely existence of a smaller group of dyslexic readers whose core deficit is in the orthographic processing and lexical knowledge domain. Second, the model will need a stronger developmental component than it now has. The developmental lag characterization of the garden-variety poor reader is a step in the right direction, but the appropriate developmental model for the dyslexic is largely unsketched. Some of the complications that elaboration of the developmental component entails have been discussed in my analysis (see Stanovich, 1986b, 1988) of Matthew effects in reading: The fact that the early acquisition of reading skill results in reading/academic experiences that facilitate the development of other cognitive structures that lay the foundation for successful reading achievement at more advanced levels. In short, there are many rich-get-richer and poor-get-poorer phenomena resulting from the interaction of the cognitive characteristics of children and their academic and home environments. I have previously outlined (see Stanovich, 1986b) how such Matthew effects can lead to a pattern where poor readers display increasingly global cognitive deficits as they get older and how early modular deficits can grow into generalized cognitive, behavioral, and motivational problems. The existence of Matthew effects raises the startling possibility that a young dyslexic might actually develop into a garden-variety poor reader! Thus, these Matthew effects complicate the prediction of the developmental growth curves for reading ability and reading-related cognitive skills, but they simply must be accounted for.

REFERENCES

Aman, M., & Singh, N. (1983). Specific reading disorders: Concepts of etiology reconsidered. In K. Gadow & I. Bialer (Eds.), *Advances in learning and behavioral disabilities* (Vol. 2, pp. 1–47). Greenwich, CT: JAI Press.

Backman, J., Bruck, M., Hebert, M., & Seidenberg, M. (1984). Acquisition and use of spelling-sound correspondences in reading. *Journal of Experimental Child Psychology, 38*, 114–133.

Baddeley, A.D., Ellis, N.C., Miles, T.R., & Lewis, V.J. (1982). Developmental and acquired dyslexia: A comparison. *Cognition, 11*, 185–199.

Baker, L.A., Decker, S.N., & DeFries, J.C. (1984). Cognitive abilities in reading-disabled children: A longitudinal study. *Journal of Child Psychology and Psychiatry, 25*, 111–117.

Baron, J., & Strawson, C. (1976). Use of orthographic and word-specific knowledge in reading words aloud. *Journal of Experimental Psychology: Human Perception and Performance, 2*, 386–393.

Baron, J., & Treiman, R. (1980). Use of orthography in reading and learning to read. In J.F. Kavanagh & R.L. Venezky (Eds.), *Orthography, reading, and dyslexia*. Baltimore: University Park Press.

Beech, J., & Harding, L. (1984). Phonemic processing and the poor reader from a developmental lag viewpoint. *Reading Research Quarterly, 19*, 357–366.

Bloom, A., Wagner, M., Reskin, L., & Bergman, A. (1980). A comparison of intellectually delayed and primary reading disabled children on measures of intelligence and achievement. *Journal of Clinical Psychology, 36*, 788–790.

Boder, E. (1973). Developmental dyslexia: A diagnostic approach based on three atypical reading-spelling patterns. *Developmental Medicine and Child Neurology, 15*, 663–687.

Bradley, L., & Bryant, P.E. (1978). Difficulties in auditory organization as a possible cause of reading backwardness. *Nature, 271*, 746–747.

Bradley, L., & Bryant, P.E. (1985). *Rhyme and reason in reading and spelling.* Ann Arbor: University of Michigan Press.

Brown, A. (1972). A rehearsal deficit in retardates' continuous short-term memory: Keeping track of variables that have few or many states. *Psychonomic Science, 29,* 373–376.

Bruck, M. (1988). The word recognition and spelling of dyslexic children. *Reading Research Quarterly, 23,* 51–69.

Bryant, P.E. & Impey, L. (1986). The similarities between normal readers and developmental and acquired dyslexics. *Cognition, 24,* 121–137.

Catts, H.W. (1986). Speech production/phonological deficits in reading-disordered children. *Journal of Learning Disabilities, 19,* 504–508.

Cohen, R.L. (1982). Individual differences in short-term memory. In N. Ellis (Ed.), *International review of research in mental retardation* (Vol. 2, pp. 43–77). New York: Academic Press.

Cohen, R.L., & Netley, C. (1981). Short-term memory deficits in reading disabled children, in the absence of opportunity for rehearsal strategies. *Intelligence, 5,* 69–76.

Cohen, R.L., Netley, C., & Clarke, M.A. (1984). On the generality of the short-term memory/reading ability relationship. *Journal of Learning Disabilities, 17,* 218–221.

Cossu, G., & Marshall, J.C. (1986). Theoretical implications of the hyperlexia syndrome: Two new Italian cases. *Cortex, 22,* 579–589.

Denckla, M.B., & Rudel, R.G. (1976). Rapid "automatized" naming (R.A.N.): Dyslexia differentiated from other learning disabilities. *Neuropsychologia, 14,* 471–479.

Dunn, L. (1965). *Peabody picture vocabulary test.* Circle Pines, MN: American Guidance Service.

Ellis, A.W. (1985). The cognitive neuropsychology of developmental (and acquired) dyslexia: A critical survey. *Cognitive Neuropsychology, 2,* 169–205.

Ellis, N., & Large, B. (1987). The development of reading: As you seek so shall you find. *British Journal of Psychology, 78,* 1–28.

Fletcher, J.M. (1981). Linguistic factors in reading acquisition. In F. Pirozzolo & M. Wittrock (Eds.), *Neuropsychology and cognitive processes in reading* (pp. 261–294). New York: Academic Press.

Fodor, J. (1983). *Modularity of mind.* Cambridge, MA: MIT Press.

Fredman, G., & Stevenson, J. (1988). Reading processes in specific reading retarded and reading backward 13-year-olds. *British Journal of Developmental Psychology, 6,* 97–108.

Gough, P.B., & Hillinger, M.L. (1980). Learning to read: An unnatural act. *Bulletin of the Orton Society, 30,* 171–176.

Gough, P.B., & Tunmer, W.E. (1986). Decoding, reading, and reading disability. *Remedial and Special Education, 7*(1), 6–10.

Hall, J., & Humphreys, M. (1982). Research on specific learning disabilities: Deficits and remediation. *Topics in Learning and Learning Disabilities, 2,* 68–78.

Hulme, C., Thompson, N., Muir, C., & Lawrence, A. (1984). Speech rate and the development of short-term memory span. *Journal of Experimental Child Psychology, 38,* 241–253.

Jackson, N.E., & Biemiller, A.J. (1985). Letter, word, and text reading times of precocious and average readers. *Child Development, 56,* 196–206.

Jorm, A. (1983). Specific reading retardation and working memory: A review. *British Journal of Psychology, 74*, 311–342.

Jorm, A., Share, D., Maclean, R., & Matthews, R. (1986). Cognitive factors at school entry predictive of specific reading retardation and general reading backward-ness: A research note. *Journal of Child Psychology and Psychiatry, 27*, 45–54.

Kavale, K., & Mattson, P. (1983). "One jumped off the balance beam": Meta-analysis of perceptual-motor training. *Journal of Learning Disabilities, 16*, 165–173.

Kochnower, J., Richardson, E., & DiBenedetto, B. (1983). A comparison of the phonic decoding ability of normal and learning disabled children. *Journal of Learning Disabilities, 16*, 348–351.

Liberman, I. (1982). A language-oriented view of reading and its disabilities. In H. Myklebust (Ed.), *Progress in learning disabilities* (Vol. 5, pp. 81–101). New York: Grune & Stratton.

Liberman, I.Y., & Shankweiler, D. (1985). Phonology and the problems of learn-ing to read and write. *Remedial and Special Education, 6*, 8–17.

Maclean, M., Bryant, P., & Bradley, L. (1987). Rhymes, nursery rhymes, and reading in early childhood. *Merrill-Palmer Quarterly, 33*, 255–281.

Manis, F.R. (1985). Acquisition of word identification skills in normal and disabled readers. *Journal of Educational Psychology, 77*, 78–90.

Mann, V. (1986). Why some children encounter reading problems. In J. Torgesen & B. Wong (Eds.), *Psychological and educational perspectives on learning disabilities* (pp. 133–159). New York: Academic Press.

McKinney, J.D. (1987). Research on the identification of learning-disabled children: Perspectives on changes in educational policy. In S. Vaughn & C. Bos (Eds.), *Research in learning disabilities* (pp. 215–233). Boston: College-Hill Press.

Morrison, F. (1984). Word decoding and rule-learning in normal and disabled readers. *Remedial and Special Education, 5*(3), 20–27.

Morrison, F.J. (1987). The nature of reading disability: Toward an integrative frame-work. In S. Ceci (Ed.), *Handbook of cognitive, social, and neuropsychological aspects of learning disabilities* (pp. 33–62). Hillsdale, NJ: Erlbaum.

Olson, R., Kliegl, R., Davidson, B., & Foltz, G. (1985). Individual and developmental differences in reading disability. In T. Waller (Ed.), *Reading research: Advances in theory and practice* (Vol. 4, pp. 1–64). London: Academic Press.

Pennington, B.F. (1986). Issues in the diagnosis and phenotype analysis of dys-lexia: Implications for family studies. In S.D. Smith (Ed.), *Genetics and learning disabilities* (pp. 69–96). San Diego: College-Hill Press.

Perfetti, C.A. (1985). *Reading ability*. New York: Oxford University Press.

Prescott, G.A., Balow, I.H., Hogan, T.P., & Farr, R.C. (1978). *Metropolitan achieve-ment tests: Survey battery*. New York: Psychological Corp.

Reynolds, C.R. (1985). Measuring the aptitude-achievement discrepancy in learn-ing disability diagnosis. *Remedial and Special Education, 6*, 37–55.

Rodgers, B. (1983). The identification and prevalence of specific reading retarda-tion. *British Journal of Educational Psychology, 53*, 369–373.

Rutter, M., & Yule, W. (1975). The concept of specific reading retardation. *Journal of Child Psychology and Psychiatry, 16*, 181–197.

Satz, P., Morris, R., & Fletcher, J.M. (1985). Hypotheses, subtypes, and individual differences in dyslexia: Some reflections. In D.B. Gray & J.F. Kavanagh (Eds.), *Biobehavioral measures of dyslexia* (pp. 25–40). Parkton, MD: New York Press.

Scarborough, H.S. (1984). Continuity between childhood dyslexia and adult reading. *British Journal of Psychology, 75*, 329–348.

Seidenberg, M.S., Bruck, M., Fornarolo, G., & Backman, J. (1985). Word recognition processes of poor and disabled readers: Do they necessarily differ? *Applied Psycholinguistics, 6*, 161–180.

Seidenberg, M.S., Bruck, M., Fornarolo, G., & Backman, J. (1986). Who is dyslexic? Reply to Wolf. *Applied Psycholinguistics, 7*, 77–84.

Share, D.L., McGee, R., McKenzie, D., Williams, S., & Silva, P.A. (1987). Further evidence relating to the distinction between specific reading retardation and general reading backwardness, *British Journal of Developmental Psychology, 5*, 35–44.

Share, D.L., McGee, R., & Silva, P.A. (in press). IQ and reading progress: A test of the "milk and jug" hypothesis. *Journal of the American Academy of Child and Adolescent Psychiatry.*

Siegel, L.S. (1985). Psycholinguistic aspects of reading disabilities. In L. Siegel & F. Morrison (Eds.), *Cognitive development in atypical children* (pp. 45–65). New York: Springer-Verlag.

Silva, P.A., McGee, R., & Williams, S. (1985). Some characteristics of 9-year-old boys with general reading backwardness or specific reading retardation. *Journal of Child Psychology and Psychiatry, 26*, 407–421.

Snowling, M. (1980). The development of grapheme-phoneme correspondence in normal and dyslexic readers. *Journal of Experimental Child Psychology, 29*, 294–305.

Snowling, M. (1981). Phonemic deficits in developmental dyslexia. *Psychological Research, 43*, 219–234.

Snowling, M., Stackhouse, J., & Rack, J. (1986). Phonological dyslexia and dysgraphia—a developmental analysis. *Cognitive Neuropsychology, 3*, 309–339.

Stanovich, K.E. (1986a). Cognitive processes and the reading problems of learning disabled children: Evaluating the assumption of specificity. In J. Torgesen & B. Wong (Eds.), *Psychological and educational perspectives on learning disabilities* (pp. 87–113). New York: Academic Press.

Stanovich, K.E. (1986b). Matthew effects in reading: Some consequences of individual differences in the acquisition of literacy. *Reading Research Quarterly, 21*, 360–407.

Stanovich, K.E. (1988). Speculations on the causes and consequences of individual differences in early reading acquisition. In P. Gough (Ed.), *Reading acquisition.* Hillsdale, NJ: Erlbaum.

Stanovich, K.E., Feeman, D.J., & Cunningham, A.E. (1983). The development of the relation between letter-naming speed and reading ability. *Bulletin of the Psychonomic Society, 21*, 199–202.

Stanovich, K.E., Nathan, R.G., & Vala-Rossi, M. (1986). Developmental changes in the cognitive correlates of reading ability and the developmental lag hypothesis. *Reading Research Quarterly, 21*, 267–283.

Stanovich, K.E., Nathan, R.G., & Zolman, J.E. (1988). The developmental lag hypothesis in reading: Longitudinal and matched reading-level comparisons. *Child Development, 59*, 71–86.

Stanovich, K.E., & West, R.F. (1983). On priming by a sentence context. *Journal of Experimental Psychology: General, 112*, 1–36.

Taylor, H.J., Satz, P., & Friel, J. (1979). Developmental dyslexia in relation to other childhood reading disorders: Significance and clinical utility. *Reading Research Quarterly, 15*, 84–101.

Torgesen, J., & Dice, C. (1980). Characteristics of research in learning disabilities. *Journal of Learning Disabilities, 13*, 531–535.

Treiman, R., & Baron, J. (1984). Individual differences in spelling: The Phoenician-Chinese distinction. *Topics in Learning and Learning Disabilities, 3*, 33–40.

Treiman, R., & Hirsh-Pasek, K. (1985). Are there qualitative differences in reading behavior between dyslexics and normal readers? *Memory and Cognition, 13*, 357–364.

Trites, R.L., & Fiedorowicz, C. (1976). Follow-up study of children with specific (or primary) reading disability. In R. Knights & D. Bakker (Eds.), *The neuropsychology of learning disorders* (pp. 41–50). Baltimore: University Park Press.

Van der Wissel, A., & Zegers, F.E. (1985). Reading retardation revisited. *British Journal of Developmental Psychology, 3*, 3–9.

Vellutino, F. (1979). *Dyslexia: Theory and research.* Cambridge, MA: MIT Press.

Wagner, R.K., & Torgesen, J.K. (1987). The nature of phonological processing and its causal role in the acquisition of reading skills. *Psychological Bulletin, 101*, 192–212.

Waters, G., Seidenberg, M., & Bruck, M. (1984). Children's and adults' use of spelling-sound information in three reading tasks. *Memory and Cognition, 12*, 293–305.

West, R.F., & Stanovich, K.E. (1978). Automatic contextual facilitation in readers of three ages. *Child Development, 49*, 717–727.

West, R.F., & Stanovich, K.E. (1982). Sources of inhibition in experiments on the effect of sentence context on word recognition. *Journal of Experimental Psychology: Learning, Memory, and Cognition, 8*, 385–399.

West, R.F., & Stanovich, K.E. (1986). Robust effects of syntactic structure on visual word processing. *Memory and Cognition, 14*, 104–112.

Williams, J. (1984). Phonemic analysis and how it relates to reading. *Journal of Learning Disabilities, 17*, 240–245.

Wolf, M. (1984). Naming, reading, and the dyslexias: A longitudinal overview. *Annals of Dyslexia, 34*, 87–115.

Zigler, E. (1969). Developmental versus difference theories of mental retardation and the problem of motivation. *American Journal of Mental Deficiency, 73*, 536–556.

3. Studies of Children with Learning Disabilities Who Perform Poorly on Memory Span Tasks

JOSEPH K. TORGESEN

Our approach to studying the cognitive characteristics of children with learning disabilities (LD) has been more narrowly focused than most. The goal of the research program reported here was to provide extensive information about the characteristics of a relatively small subgroup of children with LD. We used a clinical/rational approach to define our subgroup (Torgesen, 1982), and have thus far conducted 18 experiments designed to produce two types of information about children in the subgroup. First, we wanted to know more about their basic information processing limitations. Second, we wanted to understand how the processing limitations of children in our subgroup affect their acquisition and performance of academic skills.

We chose to study children with LD who have special difficulties with verbatim retention of relatively small amounts of information over brief periods of time. Although these children have general intellectual ability in the average range, they perform in the retarded range on tasks that require the immediate recall of sequences of items like digits, numbers, words, and letters. In the general research and clinical literature, these children are variously referred to as being deficient in short-term memory, attention span, sequencing ability, temporal perception, or auditory processing. Each of these labels implies a causal locus for the difficulties of these children on memory span tasks.

41

However, one of the major conclusions from the studies we have conducted is that none of them is an adequate characterization of the
processing difficulties of children in our subgroup.

We originally chose to study children with extreme memory span
difficulties for several reasons. First, a large body of research indicates
that children with LD, as a whole, perform poorly on memory span
tasks in comparison with children who learn normally (Heulsman, 1970;
Torgesen, 1978). At the time we began our research, the reasons for
the memory span difficulties of children with LD were not well understood. Second, performance on memory span tasks is not highly correlated with general intelligence. Traditional conceptualizations of
learning disabilities suggest that the search for LD children's special
processing limitations should begin with the abilities that are not
usually part of core definitions of general intelligence (Torgesen, 1985,
1988). The third reason we focused on children with span difficulties
came from theoretical and empirical evidence that short-term (working) memory might play an important role on some complex tasks,
but not on others (for recent reviews, see Baddeley, 1986; Crowder,
1982; Torgesen, Kistner, & Morgan, 1987). Although the memory span
task does not measure efficiency of the total working memory system
(Daneman, 1984), it is clear that memory span tasks do tap some of
the important processes that determine the functional storage capacity
of working memory (Baddeley, 1986). The final, and most practical,
reason we chose to study LD children with memory span difficulties
came from an initial survey of the records of elementary-aged children
in our local school district. This survey assured us that we could make
an initial identification of such children from existing records, and
that a sufficiently large number of children with average intelligence
was available for study.

The research described in this chapter took place over a period
of 4 years and involved studies of three different cohorts of LD children
with extreme memory span difficulties. As we identified each cohort,
we found that approximately 15% to 20% of school identified children
with LD in the fourth and fifth grades met our research criteria for
membership in the subgroup. Recently, two separate empirical
classification studies have identified subgroups of children with LD
who appear similar to the subgroup we have been studying. Lyon (1985)
found that 13% of a sample of 10- to 12-year-old children with LD
showed relatively isolated difficulties on span tasks, while an additional
23% of the students displayed these difficulties in conjunction with
more pervasive cognitive limitations. In a study of subgroups within
a sample of 59 carefully selected 9- and 10-year-old children with
reading disabilities, Speece (1987) found that 15% showed isolated
difficulties on a digit span task. An additional 20% had similar dif-

ficulties in conjunction with other processing limitations. Both of these classification studies are important to us because they place our rationally defined subgroup more precisely within the context of the LD population as a whole. They provide additional support for the idea that our conclusions apply to a significant, and reliably identifiable, subgroup of children with LD, although they are *not* applicable to the LD population as a whole.

In the remainder of this chapter, the results of our studies of LD children with memory span difficulties are summarized. The general methodology of the research is described first, followed by descriptive information concerning the severity, stability, and breadth of the children's memory difficulties. This is followed by a discussion of experiments that were designed to produce an explanation of the children's basic performance problems. Evidence showing that the processing limitations of these children affects their performance on complex academic tasks in specific ways is then provided. The chapter concludes with a brief statement about possible remedial implications and future research possibilities.

GENERAL METHODOLOGY

In all of our studies, we employed at least two control groups in addition to the target group of children with severe performance problems on span tasks. One of these control groups consisted of children with LD who were matched with target group children on age and IQ, but who did not have memory span difficulties (this group is referred to as LD-N). The second control group (N) was composed of children equivalent to the LD control group except that they were achieving at a normal rate in school.

We used five exclusionary criteria to define our subgroup of LD children with serious problems in the short-term retention of information (LD-S). First, we required all subjects to have Full Scale IQs, measured either by the Wechsler Intelligence Scale for Children–Revised (Wechsler, 1974) (WISC-R) or the Stanford-Binet (Terman & Merrill, 1960), of 85 or above. Second, the children had to be between the ages of 9 and 11 at the time they were selected. Our third criterion was that all children be at least 1.5 grade levels behind (relative to their present grade placement) in either math or reading achievement. The fourth criterion, absence of gross behavioral problems, was assessed on the basis of the psychological evaluations made on each child by school psychologists (all subjects had previously been evaluated and classified as learning disabled by an interdisciplinary team).

Our final criterion involved measurement of the central defining feature of the subgroup—their deficiencies in the short-term retention of information. We used a two-level screening procedure to select LD children with the most serious problems in this area. From information in psychological reports, we formed an initial group of children identified by school psychologists as deficient in memory span. We then individually administered the memory span task and eliminated any subjects whose variable performance on the task appeared to reflect problems in concentration or cooperation. We did not explicitly control for socioeconomic background (although the requirement for IQ above 85 almost certainly restricted our range on this variable), race, or sex of subject in our experiments, because we wanted to see if children who varied on these dimensions would have different explanations for their short-term memory problems.

In all of our experiments except one (in which an additional control group was used), we contrasted the performance of 8 LD-S children with that of 8 children in each of the other two groups (LD-N and N). Table 3.1 summarizes the characteristics of the 24 children (three separate cohorts of 8 children each) in each group that participated in our experiments over 4 years.

DESCRIPTION OF PERFORMANCE CHARACTERISTICS

In this section, we address questions concerning the severity, stability, and breadth of the memory difficulties of children in the LD-S group. In our first experiment (Torgesen & Houck, 1980, Exp 1), we established that the performance of LD-S children on span tasks was very stable over both the short and long term. The basic procedure for administration of the span test in all of our experiments involved presentation of two span trials at each length (starting with three items) until errors were made on three consecutively presented spans. A complete set of spans administered in this way is referred to as a span series. In contrast, an individual span containing a given number of items is referred to as a span trial. Span series were always presented via a tape recorder.

Short-term stability in performance was established by analyzing the between-series variability in performance across six digit span series given in one session. The performance of the LD-S group was much more stable (about 40% less variable) than that of the children in either control group. The average number of digits recalled in correct order by children in the LD-S group was 4.0, while that for the LD-N and N groups was 5.8 and 5.9, respectively. The LD-S children recalled digits about as well as normal 5- to 6-year-olds, while children in the other

TABLE 3.1
Comparison of Subject Groups on Selection Criteria

| Criteria | Subject Group | | | | | |
| | LD-S | | LD-N | | N | |
	$\overline{X}$	SD	$\overline{X}$	SD	$\overline{X}$	SD
Age (in months)	123.2	8.9	124.1	8.9	122.5	8.9
Reading (grade level)	2.6	.6	3.3	.9	5.5	1.0
Math (grade level)	3.4	.7	3.6	.7	5.2	.8
Intelligence	98.6	7.9	98.7	8.1	—[a]	—
Sex of Subject	21M	3F	22M	2F	23M	1F
Race (black or white)	16W	8B	16W	8B	17W	7B

[a]IQ scores were not available for the normal learners; however, their general achievement score on standardized tests ranged from the 35th to 65th percentile, with a mean of 54.2.

Note. LD-S = learning disabled with short-term memory deficits; LD-N = learning disabled who performed in average range on short-term memory tests; N = children with normal academic achievement.

groups performed like 9- to 12-year-olds. There were also no noticeable changes in performance on span tasks over the course of an entire year of experimentation in which the children were seen in eight sessions and experienced many trials of the span task. The results from our first experiement have been replicated many times in subsequent experiments. Whenever tasks are given that require verbatim retention of verbal items over brief periods of time, children in the LD-S group show very large and stable performance deficits.

The breadth of the memory difficulties of children in the LD-S group was addressed in a subsequent experiment (Torgesen, Rashotte, Greenstein, & Portes, 1988, Exp 2) in which nine different memory tasks were administered. These tasks included a measure of immediate recall of sequences of abstract visual forms, an incidental memory task involving recall of semantically organized information from long-term memory, two recognition memory tasks, recall of digit series in reversed order, verbatim recall of sentences, recall of digit series presented visually, and a standard aurally presented span task. Scores on each of these tasks were standardized, and they are graphically presented in Figure 3.1. The most important finding from this experiment was that children in the LD-S group did not perform poorly on all the memory tasks when compared to children in the other groups. Their performance was impaired only on tasks that specifically required the immediate verbatim recall of sequences of verbal items. On these latter tasks, it did not matter whether the items were presented visually or embedded in meaningful sentences. The relatively good perform-

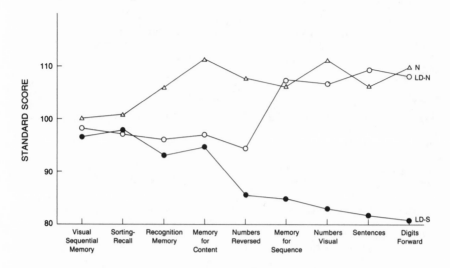

Figure 3.1.   Relative performance levels on nine different memory tasks. (LD-S = learning disabled with short-term memory deficits; LD-N = learning disabled who performed in average range on short-term memory tests; N = children with normal academic achievement.)

ance of LD-S children on the task requiring recall of meaningfully organized information is consistent with results from another experiment (Torgesen, Rashotte, & Greenstein, in press, Exp 2) in which children were required to recall the gist of interesting stories that were presented aurally. Children in the LD-S group were able to remember just as high a proportion of important idea units from these stories as children from the other groups.

To summarize, our findings thus far indicate that children in the LD-S group show substantial, and very stable, performance impairments on any task that requires short-term retention of sequences of familiar verbal information, whether presented visually or aurally. In contrast, they do not show impairments on tasks requiring the immediate recall of abstract (unfamiliar) visual information on tasks that allow semantic encoding of items or on recognition memory tasks. We turn now to experiments designed to isolate the processing disabilities underlying the performance deficits of children in the LD-S group.

INVESTIGATIONS OF PROCESSING DEFICIENCIES

There are a variety of possible explanations for performance deficits on memory span tasks (Dempster, 1981). For children with

learning disabilities, the more likely causal candidates are (a) inefficiency in the use of mnemonic strategies (Torgesen & Licht, 1983),
(b) problems coding the phonetic features of verbal information (Mann,
1986), (c) short attention span (Sattler, 1974), (d) disruptive levels of
anxiety (Hodges & Spielberger, 1969), (e) poor motivation (Hallahan,
Tarver, Kauffman, & Graybeal, 1978), or (f) problems in the perception of temporal order (Bakker, 1972). The experiments reviewed in
this section were designed to eliminate as many of these competing
hypotheses as possible in order to identify the best explanation for
the performance difficulties of children in the LD-S group.

Material incentives for better performance had no effect on the
performance of children in the LD-S group (Torgesen & Houck, 1980,
Exp 2), although they did result in a slight increase in performance
by children in both control groups. Children in the LD-S group were
as able as children in the control groups to attend to strings of digits
they did not have to recall (Torgesen & Houck, 1980, Exp 5). This result,
in combination with the information about stability of performance,
appears to rule out variable attention span as an explanation for the
memory performance problems of LD-S children. Both the relatively
good performance of LD-S children on the attention tasks and their
failure to improve in performance on span tasks as they became more
familiar and comfortable with the tasks suggest that a debilitating level
of anxiety was not a critical problem for them. Two different experiments (Torgesen et al., 1988, Exp 3; Torgesen et al., in press, Exp 3)
indicated that the short-term retention deficits of LD-S children were
not confined to sequences of information in which perception of temporal order was critical. In one experiment, children were required
to remember groups of letters without regard to order, and in the other,
they had to execute simple directions that did not have to be performed
in any particular sequence. In both cases, the relative impairment in
performance of the LD-S group was as large for nonordered recall
as for ordered recall. Thus, we do not believe that the memory span
deficits of children in the LD-S group are due to special difficulties
in sequencing information or perceiving temporal order.

Finally, the results of five experiments (Torgesen & Houck, 1980,
Exps 3, 4, & 6; Torgesen, Rashotte, Greenstein, Houck, & Portes, 1987,
Exp 1; Torgesen et al., 1988, Exp 1) combined to suggest that only a
small proportion of the performance deficits of LD-S children can be
explained by inefficiency in the use of appropriate mnemonic
strategies. Two of these experiments, for example, presented digits
at very fast rates (4 digits/sec) and found that recall differences among
groups remained the same. This finding indicates that differential use
of a strategy involving cumulative, or even isolated, rehearsal of digits
cannot explain the large performance differences between the LD-S

and other two groups. Extremely fast presentation rates effectively eliminate the possibility of such rehearsal during presentation. Further, the children were required to begin recall immediately following the last digit presented, so that use of a rehearsal strategy between presentation and recall was also effectively precluded.

One of the most widely accepted propositions about brief verbatim storage of verbal items is that it is accomplished by encoding the phonological (as opposed to the visual or semantic) features of the stimuli (Baddeley, 1986; Lachman, Lachman, & Butterfield, 1979). Thus far, we have obtained four different kinds of evidence suggesting that the performance problems of LD-S children on memory span tasks are caused by difficulties utilizing verbal/phonological codes to store information. The broadest type of evidence is the finding that these children *do not* show a performance deficit when asked to briefly retain sequences of visual figures that are difficult to label verbally (Torgesen et al., 1988, Exp 2). In other words, when information must be represented in terms of its visual features, the LD-S children performed as well as children in the control groups. This suggests that their difficulties are not the result of limitations in storage capacity per se, but rather are isolated to tasks in which information is usually represented in terms of its verbal, or phonological, features.

Verbal coding processes on short-term memory tasks are most useful when the items are familiar and have an easily accessed code available in long-term memory (Case, Kurland, & Goldberg, 1982). Our second piece of evidence concerning the coding, or representational, difficulties of children in the LD-S group comes from two experiments that have directly manipulated the familiarity of the verbal items to be coded (Torgesen & Houck, 1980, Exp 7; Torgesen et al., 1988, Exp 1). In the first of these experiments, children recalled sequences of digits, single-syllable words, and nonsense syllables. Recall of children in the two control groups was much more affected by familiarity of the items than was recall of children in the LD-S group. With totally unfamiliar verbal items (for which none of the children had an easily accessible, integrated code available in long-term memory), the recall differences were very small, but as the items became more familiar, recall differences between the LD-S and control groups became increasingly larger. In the second experiment, recall differences between groups were larger when digits (more familiar items) were used as stimuli than when letters (less familiar items) were used. These interactions between familiarity of stimuli and group performance are similar to those obtained when the performance of older and younger children are compared on span tasks (Brener, 1940; Crannel & Parrish, 1957). In both cases, the particular recall advantage of certain groups using the more familiar items can be explained in terms of their more efficient execution of coding processes for these items (Case et al., 1982; Chi, 1976).

One possible reflection of more efficient coding processes for familiar verbal items might be differences in the rate at which these items can be identified. In two experiments (Torgesen & Houck, 1980, Exp 8; Torgesen, Rashotte, Greenstein, Houck, & Portes, 1987, Exp 3), we have shown that children in the LD-S group name digits more slowly than do children in the two control groups. Although these data are not conclusive in that the rate differences were not isomorphic with span differences between the groups, they are at least consistent with the idea that children in the LD-S group have special difficulties accessing, or perhaps generating, phonological representations of verbal stimuli (Torgesen, Kistner, & Morgan, 1987).

A final piece of evidence that LD-S children have difficulties coding the phonological features of verbal stimuli comes from an experiment (Torgesen et al., 1988, Exp 4) in which we directly manipulated the distinctiveness of the phonological codes that could be used to represent information in working memory. We found that recall of children in the control groups was more affected by this manipulation than that of children in the LD-S group. That is, recall differences between groups were greatest for item sets in which the stimuli were phonologically distinct from one another, and smallest when for items that were less distinct because they rhymed with one another. This "phonological similarity effect" has been found in other experiments that have contrasted children who show strong and weak performance on span tasks (Liberman, 1987). The effect presumably occurs because children who can efficiently store verbal information in working memory can take most complete advantage of the phonetic distinctiveness between items that have little overlap in phonetic features.

When taken together, the information presented in this section converges strongly on an explanation of the performance problems of LD-S children involving difficulties utilizing phonologically based codes to store information in working memory. Since phonological codes are particularly well adapted for storage of information about the order of items as well as their identity (Drewnowski & Murdock, 1980; Salame & Baddeley, 1982), performance on a wide variety of verbatim recall tasks is affected. In fact, this processing disability should limit performance on any task that depends critically on the use of phonological codes to represent information while it is being processed. We turn now to a consideration of the effects of phonological coding deficits on complex academic tasks.

PHONOLOGICAL CODING DISABILITIES
AND ACADEMIC TASKS

Our studies of academic tasks have focused on a general examination of skills in mathematics, and a more specific examination of reading, spelling, and language comprehension skills. The data in Table 3.1 suggest that, at least on standardized measures of math skills, the children in the LD-S group are not significantly impaired when compared to LD children with other types of processing disabilities. Rather, they are deficient in reading ability when compared to their learning disabled classmates. It is no surprise that both LD groups are impaired academically when compared to nondisabled learners (they were, after all, selected from a learning disabled sample). However, the children with LD in each group were not selected because of one type of academic disability or another, so the differences between the LD groups in reading skill may reflect a special relationship between deficient phonological skills and difficulties acquiring good reading skills.

We examined the reading skills of children in the LD-S group in two experiments (Torgesen, Rashotte, Greenstein, Houck, & Portes, 1987, Exps 1 & 2). The primary finding of both experiments was that children in our target group showed special difficulties in the rapid and accurate pronunciation of individual words. In the second experiment, for example, we required children to name series of eight different digits, familiar single-syllable words, and single-syllable nonwords as rapidly and accurately as possible. They named these items in three different sessions and received intensive computer-based practice in naming the nonsense words between sessions. The naming rates from this experiment are presented in Figure 3.2. Differences in naming rate between the LD-S and control groups were significant for all three types of material, but they were particularly large for words and nonwords. This finding was explained as follows:

> If there were a real difference between LD-S and both control groups in operational efficiency of processes involved in the manipulation of phonemic codes, tasks that require children to extract multiple codes as well as perform integrative operations on them should magnify differences between groups. Both word and nonsense syllable naming undoubtedly require more processing operations on phonemic codes per item named than does digit naming. These tasks not only produced the most striking differences between the LD-S and the two control groups, but also these differences were isomorphic to differences among groups on the span task. Thus, LD-S children might have extreme difficulties on span tasks and complex naming tasks for the same reason: both kinds of tasks require them to efficiently extract and operate on multiple phonemic codes over brief periods of time. (p. 329)

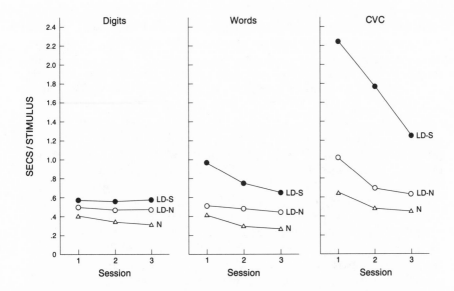

Figure 3.2. Naming rates across three sessions for digits, words, and nonsense syllables. (LD-S = learning disabled with short-term memory deficits; LD-N = learning disabled who performed in average range on short-term memory tests; N = children with normal academic achievement.) *Note.* From ''Academic Difficulties of Learning Disabled Children Who Perform Poorly on Memory Span Tasks'' by J.K. Torgesen, C.A. Rashotte, J. Greenstein, G. Houck, & P. Portes. In H.L. Swanson (Ed.), *Memory and Learning Disabilities: Advances in Learning and Behavior Disabilities,* 1987, Greenwich, CT: JAI Press. Copyright 1987 by JAI. Reprinted by permission.

This explanation implies that the phonological coding deficits of children in the LD-S group would have a particular impact during the early stages of learning to read, when words are likely to be processed as a series of separately encoded phonological elements.

Another academic task that should be sensitive to difficulties in processing the phonological components of words is learning new spelling words. In fact, children in the LD-S group had much greater difficulties on this task than did other LD children (Foster & Torgesen, 1983). The differences between LD-S and LD-N children were particularly striking when all children were required to prepare for the spelling task in an identical and systematic manner.

In contrast to their difficulties on reading and spelling tasks, children in the LD-S group performed equally well with children in the two control groups when tested on their ability to comprehend normal prose that is presented aurally. Two experiments (Torgesen et al., in press, Exps 1 & 2) have shown that, although LD-S children have difficulties remembering the specific words used to convey the meaning of passages, they do not have problems comprehending the gist of passages varying from paragraph to story length. They do have difficulties, however, in following series of directions in which the separate command segments are arbitrarily organized. These results are consistent with other research (Baddeley & Lewis, 1981; Mann, Shankweiler, & Smith, 1984) in demonstrating that only comprehension of specific types of complex prose places sufficient demands on storage processes in working memory to be affected by limitations in phonological coding efficiency. With ordinary sentence structure and passage complexity, children in the LD-S group are able to comprehend oral language as well as children in both control groups.

To summarize, the phonological coding deficiencies of children in the LD-S group appear to have their primary impact on word identification and spelling skills. Children in this group were strikingly deficient in their ability to pronounce unfamiliar, but phonologically regular, nonwords. Although children in the LD-S group were achieving significantly below grade level in math, their skills in this area were not deficient when compared to other children with LD. Finally, we were unable to discover any noticeable impact of their phonological coding deficits on comprehension of normally organized oral language.

FUTURE RESEARCH AND REMEDIAL IMPLICATIONS

Because our future research goals are closely tied to the question of appropriate remedial strategies for children in the LD-S group, these two areas are discussed together in this concluding section. We first identify some of the most important gaps in our knowledge, and then discuss potential directions for remediation.

Three broad types of questions are currently of most interest to us. First, we would like to know more about the developmental course of the processing disability manifested by children in the LD-S group. We currently have plans to conduct a 6- to 8-year follow-up of some of the children examined in the experiments reported in this paper. This follow-up will not only allow us to determine whether these children still manifest extreme deficits in phonological coding skills, but will also produce evidence about their educational prognosis relative to LD children with other types of processing disabilities. We are also interested in whether the children in our target subgroup can be identified as different from other poor readers earlier in their schooling than the fourth and fifth grades. Research reported by Liberman and colleagues (Liberman, 1987; Mann, 1986) suggests that the kinds of processing problems shown by subjects in the LD-S group may be more widespread among children in the early elementary grades. It may be the case that LD-S children would be indistinguishable from other poor readers in the first and second grades and are only unique in that they retain the processing disability while other poor readers do not. We are currently planning a longitudinal study that would measure the phonological processing skills of a large group of children in kindergarten, and then follow the subsequent development of both their academic and phonological skills over a period of several years. Such research is clearly necessary to answer questions about the relationships between children in our subgroup and other children who have difficulties learning to read.

Although we have established both theoretical and empirical links between the phonological coding deficits of children in our target subgroup and their reading difficulties, it may be that these deficits are a necessary, but not a sufficient, cause for serious reading impairment. We would also like to learn more about the broader cognitive context of these children's failure to learn to read. One strategy for doing this would be to identify, if possible, non-LD children who have similar memory deficits. Several years ago, we surveyed 350 normally achieving fourth graders and found 3 children with memory deficits as large as those of children in the LD-S group. These children had approximately normal reading skills, but they were all mildly impaired in math. We were not able to study these children extensively, or to identify more of them. However, further study of such children could determine if their memory problems were caused by processing deficits similar to those of children in the LD-S group, and, if so, help to identify circumstances or other abilities that might reduce the impact of phonological coding problems on the attainment of reading skills.

Finally, we would like to know more about the nature of the phonological coding deficit itself. One remaining question is whether the deficit is simply one of slower access to intact phonological codes, or whether slower rates of responding on item identification tasks reflect deficiencies in the codes themselves. This latter possibility is suggested in the work of Tallal (1980, in press), who has examined the ability of reading and language disabled children to discriminate rapid frequency changes in nonverbal auditory stimuli. She has shown that some poor readers (approximately 45%) have particular difficulties discriminating rapid frequency changes that occur in sequences of sounds. She has suggested that the difficulties shown on her relatively simple perceptual task might make it hard for some reading disabled children to analyze speech at the phonemic level. In a related experiment, Godfrey, Syrdal-Lasky, Millay, and Knox (1981) showed that reading disabled children were relatively inconsistent in the way they applied phonetic classifications to bits of synthetically produced speech. Both of these studies suggest that some children with LD may have subtle difficulties in the perception of speech sounds that may lead to the establishment of degraded phonetic codes for familiar verbal stimuli.

The final set of remaining questions concerns appropriate remedial procedures for children in the LD-S group. Data already available suggest some of the directions that research in this area should take. It is obvious, for example, that we should not focus directly on improving the "memory span" of these children. Although we might be able to increase their performance on span tasks by teaching them specific strategies, this would not alter the underlying coding inefficiency. In addition, the processing demands of complex tasks like decoding during reading probably preclude the allocation of conscious effort to storage activities during execution of the task (Torgesen, Kistner, & Morgan, 1987).

One way of dealing with the reading problems of children in the LD-S group is suggested in the work of Lyon (1985) with a similar subgroup of children. His preliminary studies indicated that an approach emphasizing practice in recognizing words as units was more effective with these children than one emphasizing more analytic phonetic strategies. The results of the experiment shown in Figure 3.2 are consistent with Lyon's findings. That is, the special improvement in nonword reading that occurred for the LD-S group as the result of intensive practice probably reflected the formation of more unitized (Ehri & Wilce, 1983) codes for the stimuli they were required to read. The differences between the LD-S and control groups in naming rate for nonwords declined as all children began to process the nonwords more like digits; in terms of a single, unitized code. These findings suggest that children in the LD-S group may have special needs for practice sequences in reading that use speed of response as a criterion for lesson mastery, since speed of response is probably the best indicator that recognition of words as whole units has been achieved. One approach we have been experimenting with is the use of computers (Torgesen, 1986) to provide decoding practice that focuses on several different levels of word representation during reading.

Another approach to remediation for children in the LD-S group would involve explicit instruction and practice in identifying the phonological structure of speech. Several studies with younger children (Bradley & Bryant, 1985; Williams, 1980) have shown that such instruction can have positive effects on the acquisition of decoding skills in reading. Although we have not directly tested the possibility, children in the LD-S group may be less aware of the phonological structure of words than children with better developed phonological processing skills (Bradley & Bryant, 1978; Wagner & Torgesen, 1987). If this is the case, then intensive training in the phonemic analysis of speech might help them apply analytic decoding skills more effectively.

REFERENCES

Baddeley, A.D. (1986). *Working memory.* New York: Oxford University Press.

Baddeley, A.D. & Lewis, V. (1981). Inner active processes in reading: The inner voice, the inner ear, and the inner eye. In A.M. Lesgold & C.A. Perfetti (Eds.), *Interactive processes in reading* (pp. 107–129). Hillsdale NJ: Erlbaum.

Bakker, D.J. (1972). *Temporal order in disturbed reading.* Rotterdam, The Netherlands: Rotterdam University.

Bradley, L., & Bryant, P.E. (1978). Difficulties in auditory organization as a possible cause of reading backwardness. *Nature, 221,* 746–747.

Bradley, L., & Bryant, P. (1985). *Rhyme and reason in reading and spelling.* Ann Arbor: University of Michigan Press.

Brener, R. (1940). An experimental investigation of memory span. *Journal of Experimental Psychology, 26,* 467–482.

Case, R., Kurland, D.M., & Goldberg, L. (1982). Operational efficiency and the growth of short-term memory span. *Journal of Experimental Child Psychology, 33,* 386–404.

Chi, M.T. (1976). Short term memory limitations in children: Capacity or processing deficits? *Memory and Cognition, 4,* 559–572.

Crannel, C.W., & Parrish, J.M. (1957). A comparison of immediate memory span for digits, letters, and words. *Journal of Psychology, 44,* 319–327.

Crowder, R.C. (1982). *The psychology of reading.* New York: Cambridge University Press.

Daneman, M. (1984). Why some people are better readers than others: A process and storage account. In R.J. Stennberg (Ed.), *Advances in the psychology of human intelligence* (pp. 367–384). Hillsdale, NJ: Erlbaum.

Dempster, F.N. (1981). Memory span sources of individual and developmental differences. *Psychological Bulletin, 89,* 63–100.

Drewnowski, A., & Murdock, B. (1980). The role of auditory features in memory span for words. *Journal of Experimental Psychology: Human Learning and Memory, 6,* 315–332.

Ehri, L., & Wilce, L. (1983). Development of word identification speed in skilled and less skilled beginning readers. *Journal of Educational Psychology, 75,* 3–18.

Foster, K., & Torgesen, J.K. (1983). The effects of directed study on the spelling performance of two subgroups of learning disabled children. *Learning Disability Quarterly, 6,* 252–257.

Godfrey, J.J., Syrdal-Lasky, A.K., Millay, K.K., & Knox, C.M. (1981). Performance of dyslexic children on speech perception tests. *Journal of Experimental Child Psychology, 32,* 401–424.

Hallahan, D.P., Tarver, S.G., Kauffman, J.M., & Graybeal, N.L. (1978). Selective attention abilities of learning disabled children under reinforcement and response cost. *Journal of Learning Disabilities, 11,* 42–51.

Heulsman, C.B. (1970). The WISC subtest syndrome for disabled readers. *Perceptual and Motor Skills, 30,* 535–550.

Hodges, W., & Spielberger, C. (1969). Digit span: An indicant of trait or state anxiety? *Journal of Consulting and Clinical Psychology, 33,* 430–434.

Lachman, R., Lachman, J.L., & Butterfield, E.C. (1979). *Cognitive psychology and information processing.* Hillsdale, NJ: Erlbaum.

Liberman, I.Y. (1987). Language and literacy: The obligation of the schools of education. In R.F. Bowler (Ed.), *Intimacy with language* (pp. 1–9). Baltimore: The Orton Dyslexia Society.

Lyon, G.R. (1985). Educational validation studies. In B.P. Rourke (Ed.), *Neuropsychology of learning disabilities* (pp. 228–253). New York: Guilford.

Mann, V.A. (1986). Why some children encounter reading problems: The contribution of difficulties with language processing and phonological sophistication to early reading disability. In J.K. Torgesen & B.Y.L. Wong (Eds.), *Psychological and educational perspectives on learning disabilities* (pp. 133–160). New York: Academic Press.

Mann, V.A., Shankweiler, D., & Smith, S.T. (1984). The association between comprehension of spoken sentences and early reading ability: The role of phonetic representation. *Journal of Child Language, 11,* 627–643.

Salame, P., & Baddeley, A. (1982). Disruption of short-term memory by unattended speech: Implications for the structure of working memory. *Journal of Verbal Learning and Verbal Behavior, 21,* 150–164.

Sattler, J.M. (1974). *Assessment of children's intelligence.* Philadelphia: Saunders.

Speece, D.L. (1987). Information processing subtypes of learning disabled readers. *Learning Disabilities Research, 2,* 91–102.

Tallal, P. (1980). Auditory temporal perception, phonics, and reading disabilities in children. *Brain and Language, 9,* 182–198.

Tallal, P. (in press). Developmental language disorders. In J.F. Kavanagh & T. Truss (Eds.), *Proceedings of the National Conference on Learning Disabilities.* Bethesda, MD: National Institutes of Health.

Terman, L.M., & Merrill, M.A. (1960). *Stanford-Binet intelligence scale: Form L-M.* Boston: Houghton Mifflin.

Torgesen, J.K. (1978). Performance of reading disabled children on serial memory tasks: A review. *Reading Research Quarterly, 19,* 57–87.

Torgesen, J.K. (1982). The use of rationally defined subgroups in research on learning disabilities. In J.P. Das, R.F. Mulcahy, & A.E. Wells (Eds.), *Theory and research in learning disabilities* (pp. 111–132). New York: Plenum Press.

Torgesen, J.K. (1985). Memory processes in reading disabled children. *Journal of Learning Disabilities, 18,* 350–357.

Torgesen, J.K. (1986). Practicing reading on computers: A research based perspective. *Learning Disabilities Focus, 1,* 72–81.

Torgesen, J.K. (1988). Applied research and metatheory in the context of contemporary cognitive theory. *Journal of Learning Disabilities, 21,* 271–274.

Torgesen, J.K., & Houck, G. (1980). Processing deficiencies in learning disabled children who perform poorly in the digit span task. *Journal of Educational Psychology, 72,* 141–160.

Torgesen, J.K., Kistner, J.A., & Morgan, S. (1987). Component processes in working memory. In J. Borkowski & J.D. Day (Eds.), *Memory and cognition in special children: Perspectives on retardation, learning disabilities, and giftedness*. Norwood, NJ: Ablex.

Torgesen, J.K., & Licht, B. (1983). The learning disabled child as an inactive learner: Retrospect and prospects. In J.D. McKinney & L. Feagans (Eds.), *Topics in learning disabilities* (Vol. 1, pp. 3–32). Rockville, MD: Aspen.

Torgesen, J.K., Rashotte, C.A., & Greenstein, J. (in press). Language comprehension in learning disabled children who perform poorly on memory span tests. *Journal of Educational Psychology*.

Torgesen, J.K., Rashotte, C.A., Greenstein, J., Houck, G., & Portes, P. (1987). Academic difficulties of learning disabled children who perform poorly on memory span tasks. In H.L. Swanson (Ed.), *Memory and learning disabilities: Advances in learning and behavioral disabilities* (pp. 305–333). Greenwich, CT: JAI.

Torgesen, J.K., Rashotte, C.A., Greenstein, J., & Portes, P. (1988). *Further studies of learning disabled children who perform poorly on memory span tests*. Unpublished manuscript, Florida State University, Tallahassee.

Wagner, R.K., & Torgesen, J.K. (1987). The nature of phonological processing and its causal role in the acquisition of reading skills. *Psychological Bulletin, 101,* 192–212.

Wechsler, D. (1974). *Wechsler intelligence scale for children–Revised.* New York: Psychological Corp.

Williams, J.P. (1980). Teaching decoding with an emphasis on phoneme analysis and phoneme blending. *Journal of Educational Psychology, 72,* 1–15.

4. Phonological Processing, Language Comprehension, and Reading Ability

VIRGINIA A. MANN, ELIZABETH COWIN,

AND JOYCE SCHOENHEIMER

What makes a poor reader a poor *reader*? There are many reasons why a child might fail to read well, for the act of reading recruits a variety of cognitive abilities that spread between the domains of visual skills and language skills. In the past, many educators and research scientists focused their studies of reading disability on the visual requirements of reading and sought to blame reading problems on some disability in the visual domain. However, there is little support for this conjecture, for careful scientific research has shown that children deficient in visual-motor and/or visual-perceptual skills do not encounter reading difficulty any more frequently than do matched controls (Robinson & Schwartz, 1973). Even the reversal errors that were once regarded as a hallmark of dyslexia seem to be common to all young children (Mann, Tobin, & Wilson, 1987; Simner, 1982) and not a true cause of children's reading errors (Fischer, Liberman, & Shankweiler,

The research reported in this paper was conducted at Bryn Mawr College, supported primarily by NICHD Grant No. HD211-82-01 to the senior author. Preparation of this manuscript has been partially funded by NICHD Grant No. HDO1994 to Haskins Laboratories, Inc. We would like to thank Judith Berman for her help in developing the test materials and in pilot research.

1977). Thus there is general consensus in the field that only a few instances of reading difficulty can be traced to a difficulty in visual processing (cf. Rayner, 1985; Stanovich, 1985; Vellutino, 1979).

Rather than being visually based, many instances of reading difficulty appear to be language based. Research on the relationship between reading problems and memory problems offers one example of a domain in which language-based processes offer a compelling account of the differences between good and poor readers. A clear demonstration of this point is offered by a study in which good and poor beginning readers who were equated for age and IQ were asked to remember various types of visual stimuli (Liberman, Mann, Shankweiler, & Werfelman, 1982). The poor readers were equivalent to the good readers in their memory for nonlinguistic visual material— faces of strangers and nonsense doodle drawings—refuting any claim that they suffered from a basic problem with visual memory, or some generalized memory impairment. Yet when they were asked to remember linguistic visual material—printed nonsense syllables—these same children made significantly more errors than the good readers. Further research has shown other linguistic memory problems among poor readers, and these are not limited to visual linguistic material; they spread to spoken material as well. Not only do poor readers have difficulty remembering spoken nonsense words (Brady, Mann, & Schmidt, 1987), but they also fail to remember spoken words as well as good readers, even when these words form meaningful sentences (Mann, Liberman, & Shankweiler, 1980).

The linguistic memory tasks that distinguish poor readers from the better readers of their classrooms have in common a demand on working memory (sometimes referred to as short-term memory). In this chapter we develop the view that a limited ability to hold linguistic material in short-term memory is one aspect of a phonological processing problem, and we report a set of two experiments that show how this limitation can lead poor readers to misunderstand certain types of phrases and sentences. The first experiment compares good and poor readers' ability to understand phrases and sentences that place considerable demands on the ability to remember and interpret the phonological structure (i.e., the sound structure) of language. The discovery in the first experiment that poor readers make more comprehension errors than good readers led to the second experiment, which asks whether misunderstanding reflects poor perception or poor memory. Both experiments were designed to shed light on the question of why poor readers have a language problem in the first place. The particular explanation that we shall consider is a maturational account: Many poor readers may be delayed in their development of certain language skills.

PHONOLOGICAL PROCESSING:
A PROBLEM FOR POOR READERS

There is much evidence that reading problems in the early elementary grades often stem from a problem with spoken language that can be characterized as a phonological processing deficiency. Evidence of this deficiency stems from a variety of sources. For example, poor beginning readers make more errors than good beginning readers of the same age in perceiving speech in noise (Brady, Shankweiler, & Mann, 1983), in repeating sequences of spoken words, and in repeating spoken sentences (Holmes & McKeever, 1979; Jorm, 1979, 1983; Mann et al., 1980; McKeever & Van Deventer, 1975). They also tend to comprehend certain types of spoken sentences less accurately, although they make the same types of errors that better readers do (Mann, Shankweiler, & Smith, 1984; Smith, Mann, & Shankweiler, 1987). In all of the above-mentioned cases, the inferior performance of the poorer readers cannot be attributed to basic auditory deficits, attentional deficits, deficient intelligence, a general memory impairment, and so forth, so much as to some type of language impairment. This accords with other findings that measures of spoken language skill tend to be stronger associates of early reading skill than visual skills, intelligence, or other general cognitive abilities (for a review, see Jorm & Share, 1983; Liberman, 1983; Mann, 1984a, 1986; Stanovich, Cunningham, & Freeman, 1984).

Many of the tasks that distinguish good and poor readers require effective processing of the sound elements of language and the regular patterns among them, which is to say that they require effective processing of the phonological structure of spoken language (for discussion, see Jorm & Share, 1983; Liberman & Mann, 1980; Mann, 1986; Wagner & Torgesen, 1987). Even the poor readers' problems with sentence comprehension may be rooted in a phonological processing limitation, for it is primarily those sentences and test procedures that stress phonological working memory that have distinguished poor readers from good readers of the same age. Hence it may not be insufficient grammatical knowledge (i.e., linguistic competence) so much as poor processing skills that lead poor readers to make more errors than good readers on language comprehension tasks (see Shankweiler & Crain, 1986). Evidence that this is the case has been offered by several studies showing that poor readers understand the same types of structures that good readers do, and have difficulty with the same structures that are difficult for other children—they merely make more of the same kinds of errors, especially when the test materials or the testing paradigm places inordinate demands on the child's ability to hold the sentence in working memory. These demands can arise in the comprehension of relative clause sentences (e.g., *The cat jumped over the dog that chased the turtle*) and Token test instructions that contain several confusable adjectives (e.g., *Touch the small red triangle and the large blue square*), and are exacerbated by testing situations where the child must act out the meaning of a lengthy sentence (see Mann et al., 1984; Smith, 1987; Smith, Mann & Shankweiler, 1986).

To corroborate the association between poor reading, inadequate phonological processing skills, and poor language comprehension, we conducted an experiment that considers the relation between children's reading ability and their comprehension of utterances that stress the use of prosodic cues. Prosodic cues are an aspect of phonological structure that has received little attention in previous research. They are critical markers of sentence meaning and can offer an excellent probe to the association between phonological processing and language comprehension. Previous research (to be discussed below) has shown age-related differences in children's comprehension of prosodic cues, and these developmental differences can be used to test a maturational account of the differences between good and poor readers. According to a maturational account, reading-ability-related differences in phonological processing skills might be due to individual differences in the rate at which those skills develop (see Mann & Liberman, 1984, and Mann, 1986, for a discussion). If this view is correct, then the differences between good and poor readers should parallel those between older and younger children, and the performance of poor readers should resemble that of younger children who are reading at their same level.

EXPERIMENT 1

By definition, prosodic cues are an aspect of phonological structure that include the melodic (i.e., pitch) contour of an utterance, as well as any differences in the amplitude and duration of individual words and the pauses between them. They can assist the listeners' recovery of the grammatical structure of phrases and sentences because they mark word class and the boundaries between and within phrases and sentences. There has been some speculation that prosodic cues might pose a particular problem for poor readers, as "supersegmental" relations that span several phonetic segments might stress the ability to hold phonetic information in working memory (as suggested by Shankweiler & Liberman, 1976).

Age-related changes in the use of prosodic cues are intimated by certain findings about children's sentence comprehension abilities. Although some sensitivity to prosodic cues is present in early infancy (see Gleitman & Wanner, 1982, for a discussion), children below age 10 may not comprehend prosodic cues as well as adults. For example, when sentences like 1A and 1B are spoken, the prosodic cues of pitch, stress, and pause supplement the location of the definite article (*the*) as markers of the boundary between the indirect and direct object.

1A He showed [her baby] [the pictures].
 B He showed [her] [the baby pictures].

Using such cues, a speaker may omit the definite article and still be able to convey his or her intended meaning to adult listeners (as noted by Scholes, Tanis, & Turner, 1976). However, children below age 10 are prone to confuse 1A and 1B, in general, and those nearing age 10 are particularly dependent upon the presence of the article (Scholes et al., 1976). Scholes et al. (1976) suggest that children's difficulty with these sentences reflects insufficient knowledge of a particular grammatical structure—the double object construction. Yet there are some other observations that even very young children (i.e., those in Stage 1 of language development) produce sentences with double object constructions (see Pinker, 1984, for a discussion of the relevant data). Early production implies that insufficient knowledge of grammar cannot explain children's tendency to confuse 1A and 1B, and leaves room for other explanations such as Pinker's (1984) suggestion that double object constructions are difficult for children to comprehend because they are difficult to parse. We suggest that children know about the double object construction but have some difficulty recovering the structure of sentences like 1A and 1B because to do so requires effective use of prosodic cues.

This logic led us to compare good and poor readers' comprehension of sentences like 1A and 1B, predicting that the deficient phonological processing skills of poor readers may lead them to problems in distinguishing 1A and 1B. However, since it is always desirable to guard against some type of material-specific effect, we also examined the comprehension of noun phrases like those in 2A and 2B:

2A big green // house
 B big // greenhouse

As compared to the sentences in 1A and 1B, these materials are shorter and contain less syntactic embedding, yet they still exploit prosodic cues. Indeed, such cues are the only markers of constituent structure. We would not expect that the syntactic structure of these noun phrases would pose any difficulty for school-aged children, given what is known of children's comprehension of noun phrases that consist of one or more adjectives modifying a noun. Matthei (1982) has reported that children from 4 to 5 years make more errors than adults on phrases like "second green ball" because they tend to "flatten" embedded structures, but such flattening should not interfere with comprehension of 2A versus 2B. Also, Hamburger and Crain (1984) have presented evidence that children's flattening errors are not due to insufficient structural knowledge about embedded clauses so much as to problems in formulating and executing a plan of action. More pointedly, Smith et al. (1987) have found that neither good nor poor readers make many errors when asked to execute commands like "Touch the small red circle." Differences between the two groups emerge only in the case of sentences like "Touch the small red circle and the large green square," which contain the same structure but are considerably longer and require the selection/touching of two items, each marked by two adjectives. So, all in all, there is little reason to think that this noun phrase structure should cause any problem for either young children or poor readers.

A previous study of good and poor readers has already noted significant differences in children's comprehension of sentences like 1A and 1B (Fletcher, Satz, & Scholes, 1981). However, instead of concentrating on prosodic cues, as such, that study concentrated on the possibility that poor readers suffer from a delay in the development of language skills, and illustrated the value of a maturational account. We decided to ask whether we could interrelate our phonological processing account with the maturational account of poor readers' problems with sentence comprehension. Accordingly, we chose to test children at two different ages, second and fourth grade, so as to determine whether any differences between the good and poor readers run parallel to those between younger and older children (as opposed to representing a true deviance). Such a parallel would suggest that good and poor readers occupy different positions along some developmental continuum.

As another test of the maturational account, we ask whether poor readers in the fourth grade are equivalent to younger children who are reading at the same level. Recently, the use of such reading-ability-matched (RAM) controls has been advocated as a means of establishing whether differences between age-matched good and poor readers are a consequence of differences in written language experience rather than their cause (Backman, Mamen, & Ferguson, 1984; Bryant & Goswami, 1986). Our focus on spoken language comprehension helps to circumvent some of the problems of causality, but we may still profit from use of a RAM control group as a direct test of the maturational delay theory of reading difficulty (as did Stanovich, Nathan, & Valla-Rossi, in press).

METHOD

Subjects

The available population of children included 57 second graders and 57 fourth graders, all of whom were rated by their reading teacher as good (one or more grades above level), high average (between one-half and one grade above level), average, low average (between one-half and one grade below level), or poor (one or more grades below level) in reading ability. This rating established 10 good readers in the second grade (4 boys and 6 girls), 9 poor readers in the second grade (6 boys and 3 girls), 12 good readers in the fourth grade (6 boys and 6 girls), and 9 poor readers in the fourth grade (7 boys and 2 girls).

The children in this study were not selected according to IQ; thus the poor readers are of the garden-variety type discussed by Stanovich (1988). To confirm that the subjects did, indeed, differ in reading ability, we administered the word identification and word attack subtests of the Woodcock Reading Mastery Test (Woodcock, 1973). The good and poor readers were found to differ significantly in the accuracy of word identification: 119 versus 74 for second graders, $t(17) = 8.76$, $p < .000$, and 136 versus 105 for fourth graders, $t(19) = 12.07$, $p < .000$. They also differed in word attack: 41 versus 13 for second graders, $t(17) = 8.80$, $p < .000$, and 49 versus 32 for fourth graders, $t(19) = 6.19$, $p < .000$.

Based on the results of the Woodcock test, a fifth group of subjects was formed by selecting second graders who were reading-ability-matched (RAM) controls for the fourth-grade poor readers. Each poor reader in the fourth-grade sample was matched with an average reader in the second grade who had achieved the same word identification score (within 4 points) on the Woodcock test. This yielded a group of 9 children whose mean reading scores were not significantly different from those of the fourth-grade poor readers on either the word identification test (mean score 105.4, $t(16) = 0.13$, $p > .897$) or the word attack test (mean score 36.1, $t(16) = 1.05$, $p > .308$).

In preparing the materials, we also made use of 10 college students who served as paid volunteers. These subjects made less than 5% errors in comprehension of the test materials.

Materials

Two comprehension tests were administered, a sentence comprehension test and a noun phrase comprehension test. Both involved spoken materials that had been prerecorded in a fixed random order in a natural speaking voice by a female native speaker of English. Comprehension was measured with a four-alternative, forced-choice picture verification procedure, a procedure in which children listened to an item and chose its illustration from among an array of four numbered line drawings. Each array included an illustration of the item at hand, an illustration of the likely misinterpretation (i.e., the other member of its minimal pair), and the two illustrations of another (irrelevant) minimal pair of items. A separate array was prepared for each item, and the positions of the correct response and the various foils were systematically varied across items.

For the Sentence Comprehension Test, the items were constructed from six minimal pairs of sentences like those illustrated in 1A and 1B above, three of which had been taken from Scholes, Tanis, and Turner (1976). Each pair of sentences was used to construct four different items, by presenting each sentence version (A or B) with or without the article (+ Article or − Article). This yielded a total of 24 test items (6 pairs × 2 versions × 2 forms of presentation). Pilot testing revealed an extremely high rate of accuracy; across the 10 adult subjects whom we tested, only a single error was made on one of the A, − Article items.

For the Noun Phrase Comprehension Test, the stimuli included six minimal pairs of noun phrases like those illustrated in 2A and 2B above. There was a total of 12 items (6 pairs × 2 versions), and pilot testing revealed the adults to be 100% accurate in the comprehension of each item.

Procedure

Children were tested in groups of 15 to 30 in a single session that lasted approximately 30 minutes. The sentence test was given at the onset of the session, followed by the noun phrase test. All materials were presented over a loudspeaker at a comfortable listening level; subjects were told that they would be hearing some sentences and were given test booklets from which to choose the picture that showed the meaning of each sentence. They recorded the number of the picture (1 to 4) on the response sheet.

RESULTS

Performance on the two tests was significantly correlated, $r(40) = .54$, $p < .01$, and on both tests the younger children and the poorer readers tended to make more errors than the older children and the better readers. It was also the case that the fourth-grade poor readers made the same number of errors as the second graders who were reading at the same level.

The Sentence Comprehension Test

To analyze the results of this test we computed four accuracy scores for each child, summing across the six sentence tokens but maintaining the orthogonal variation in version (A or B) and form of presentation (+ Article or − Article). Figure 4.1 summarizes the mean percentage of correct responses to each type of item according to children's age and reading ability. In that figure it can be seen that more errors had been made by poor readers, $F(1,36) = 30.13, p < .000$ (MSE = 16.56), and by younger children, in general, $F(1,36) = 27.85, p < .000$ (MSE = 15.31).

As noted by Scholes and his colleagues, all children made fewer errors on the B version (i.e., the version where the direct object was a compound noun), $F(1,36) = 47.93, p < .000$ (MSE = 29.78). Like Scholes et al. (1976), we find this effect to be stronger in younger subjects, $F(1,36) = 8.31, p < .007$ (MSE = 5.16). We also find the effect of sentence version to be stronger for poor readers, $F(1,36) = 25.3, p < .000$ (MSE = 15.72). When the article was omitted from the test sentences, we found, as did Scholes and his colleagues, that all children made more errors, $F(1,36) = 16.41, p < .001$ (MSE = 6.03), especially on the A versions, $F(1,36) = 9.39, p < .004$ (MSE = 3.34). Scholes et al. also reported this effect to be particularly strong for older children, but we failed to replicate this result (possibly because we studied a narrower age range). Likewise, the extent of differences between good and poor readers was not a function of the presence versus absence of the article. All other interactions were nonsignificant $(p > .1)$.

Comparison of the fourth-grade poor readers and their reading-ability-matched controls reveals that they performed equivalently in all respects. Both groups of children were more accurate on the B versions, $F(1,16) = 21.69, p < .000$ (MSE = 22.22), when the article is present, $F(1,16) = 5.56, p < .006$ (MSE = 5.56), and these effects interact, $F(1,16) = 9.82, p < .006$ (MSE = 5.56). However, the older poor readers and their RAM controls did not differ in their susceptibility to any of these effects, or in overall performance $(p > .1)$.

The Noun Phrase Comprehension Test

To analyze the results of this test we computed two accuracy scores, summing across the six tokens of each version (A vs. B). The results

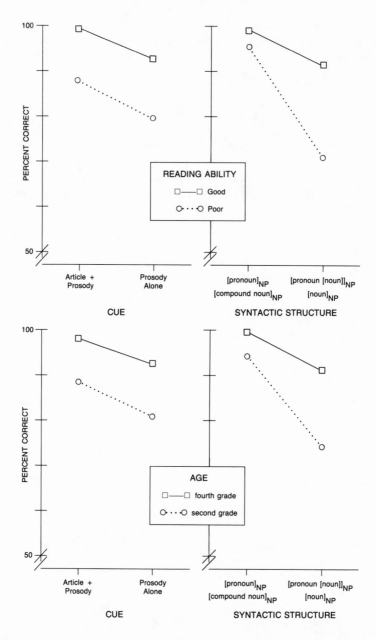

Figure 4.1. The parallel effects of reading ability and age on children's sentence comprehension. For test materials like those in examples 1A and 1B, the effects of reading appear in the top two panels; those of age appear in the bottom two panels. The left-hand panels contrast sentences in which an article was or was not present, whereas the right-hand ones compare those that contained a compound noun (i.e., *birdseed*) with those that contained a simple noun (i.e., *seed*).

appear in Figure 4.2, where it may be seen that the poorer readers, $F(1,36) = 28.63$, $p < .000$ (MSE = 36.69), and the younger children, $F(1,36) = 12.08$, $p < .001$ (MSE = 15.49), made more errors than the better readers and the older children. There was no main effect of version, and no interactions. Finally, the fourth-grade poor readers and their RAM controls performed at the same level ($p > .1$) and were equally unaffected by version ($p > .1$).

DISCUSSION

Consistent with previous indications of a relationship between reading ability and language comprehension, this experiment has revealed that poor readers made more errors than good readers on two different tests of spoken language comprehension. Each test presented a grammatical structure that should be well within the grasp of all of our subjects; hence performance differences are not likely to reflect inadequate knowledge of grammar so much as some difficulty with using that knowledge. Each test was designed to make critical demands on the ability to use prosodic cues in the recovery of grammatical structure, and this demand is a candidate source of the differences between good and poor readers.

According to a maturational account of the differences between good and poor readers, we would have expected poor readers to resemble younger children, whereas good readers would resemble older children. The data from both tests meet this prediction, as does the observation that the fourth-grade poor readers performed at the same level as a group of RAM controls on both tests. These parallels are not likely to be trivial consequences of the fact that older children and good readers have had more written language experience than younger children and poor readers, since the test materials did not manipulate cues that are systematically marked in written language. We suggest that the parallels between good versus poor readers and older versus younger children may not reflect differences in written language experience so much as differences in the maturation of certain phonological processing skills.

Two aspects of the sentence comprehension data could challenge an account that stresses the role of prosodic cues as opposed to the role of grammatical knowledge. One is the fact that the extent of differences between good and poor readers, younger and older children, remained the same whether or not an article was present at the site of the boundary between the direct and indirect object. If poor comprehension reflects some difficulty with prosodic cues, shouldn't com-

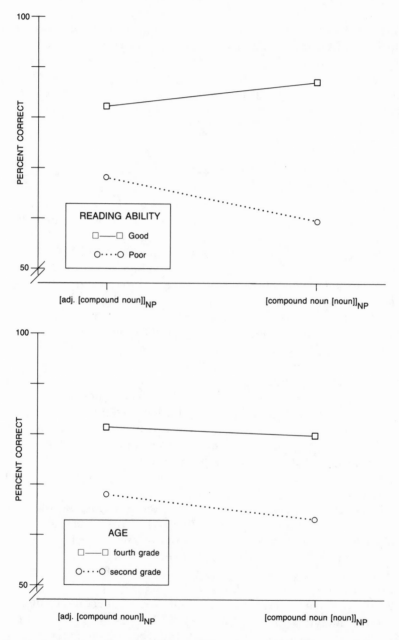

Figure 4.2. The parallel effects of reading ability and age on children's comprehension of noun phrases. For test materials like those in examples 2A and 2B, the effects of reading ability appear in the top panel; those of age are on the bottom. Each panel contrasts phrases that ended in a compound noun (i.e., *black birdfeeder*) with those that ended in a simple noun (i.e., *blackbird feeder*).

prehension have been at its worst when prosodic cues were the only cue at stake? Perhaps the omission of the article decreased demands on working memory at the same time as it increased demands on the use of prosodic cues—a reduced demand on memory resources may have made poor readers/younger children more capable of using the prosodic cues in our test materials and thereby more tolerant of the stress on those cues. This line of reasoning assumes that poor readers and younger children might be capable of using prosodic cues, in principle, but are prevented from doing so by a processing limitation. We offer a test of this possibility in Experiment 2.

A second challenge comes from the findings about the significant effect of sentence version: The poor readers and younger children tended to favor the "compound noun" interpretation (i.e., sentence 1B) more strongly than good readers and older children. Scholes et al. (1976) noted a similar bias, which they attributed to insufficient knowledge of the double object construction. However, as we noted earlier, this interpretation is at odds with other evidence that young children produce the double object construction quite early in language development. Moreover, a conclusion that poor readers lack knowledge of this construction is at odds with some other data (presented in Shankweiler, Smith, & Mann, 1984) that poor readers equal good readers in the comprehension of the pronoun in sentences like *The girl made her a sandwich* versus *The girl made herself a sandwich*.

In other studies of sentence comprehension and reading ability, it has been noted that problems with phonological processing skills may lead poor readers to parse sentences "as if" they lack structural knowledge (see Shankweiler & Crain, 1986). One such case has been documented in a recent doctoral thesis by Smith (1987), who studied good and poor readers' comprehension of relative clause structures, which a previous study (Mann et al., 1984) had shown to be a particular problem for poor readers. Smith observed that by decreasing the memory demands of test items and by changing the procedure from toy manipulation to picture verification, poor readers could be made to perform as well as good readers. Hence it was not the relative clause structure, as such, that caused the poor readers to make more errors; it was the demands on working memory that arose from sentence length and the toy manipulation procedure (as Mann et al., 1984; Shankweiler et al., 1984; and Shankweiler & Crain, 1986, had suggested).

Such observations lead us to speculate that constraints on working memory, perception, or some other aspect of phonological processing may have led poor readers (and maybe all younger children) to show a "compound noun" bias, "as if" they lack appropriate syntactic knowledge. To test this possibility, Experiment 2 probes the effects of disrupted prosodic structure on children's comprehension.

Subjects who normally make use of prosodic cues should make significantly more errors when prosodic cues are disrupted, whereas those who make less effective use of prosodic cues should be more tolerant of the disruption.

If prosodic cues pose a problem for poor readers and younger children, then their perception of prosodic cues could be faulty. Perhaps these children cannot perceive subtle differences in pitch, stress, and so forth. Accordingly, Experiment 2 also asks whether good and poor readers, older and younger children, are equally capable of perceiving the prosodic cues that were present in the test sentences. It asks children to discriminate nonsense utterances that contrast the prosodic cues at stake in Experiment 1. It also attempts to boost the performance of the poor readers/younger children by making the juncture pause twice as long, following a speculation by Scholes et al. (1976) that performance of younger children is limited by poor perception of the juncture pause at the site of the boundary between the direct and indirect object.

Even if perception were intact, problems with holding phonological information in memory could lead to difficulty in using prosodic cues in order to recover syntactic structure (as suggested by Shankweiler & Liberman, 1976). For this reason, Experiment 2 asks whether the poor readers who participated in Experiment 1 do, indeed, possess a phonological processing difficulty in linguistic working memory. It further asks whether linguistic working memory ability is related to poor comprehension in Experiment 1 prosodic cues and whether memory differences between good and poor readers find a parallel in the behavior of older versus younger children. To confirm that any memory deficit is limited to the language domain, we also assess temporary memory for visual-spatial sequences.

EXPERIMENT 2

METHOD

Subjects

Experiment 2 included the same subjects who participated in Experiment 1: the five groups of children, and a new group of 26 college students.

Materials

Sentence Comprehension Materials.   The materials were 40 test sentences constructed from a subset of the sentences employed in Experiment 1: The A, – Article and B, – Article versions of five minimal pairs of sentences were digitized at 10000Hz and manipulated with a wave-form editor to form four different forms of each sentence (5 pairs × 2 versions × 4 forms). The control form (C) left the original version intact. The emphasized pause form (EP) attempted to facilitate interpretation by making the juncture pause 350 msec longer than normal. (Measures of the test items had indicated that the average duration of that pause was 367 msec; accordingly, each pause was increased by 350 msec.) The remaining two forms disrupted prosodic cues by pitting word stress and juncture pause against each other (these being the major cues at stake in adults' perception of phrase boundary location; see Grosjean, Grosjean, & Lane, 1979; Streeter, 1978). The transposed pause form (TP) decreased the pause at the clause boundary to 50 msec (47 msec was the average duration of the pause at the alternative site, and is commensurate with normal stop consonant closure duration), and increased the pause at the alternative location (i.e., the location of the boundary in the other version of the core pair) by 300 msec. The transposed stress form (TS) excised and transposed the last words of the A-P and B-P forms of each core pair. By transposing the final words, we effectively disrupted the stress contour of the test items and rendered stress an ineffective cue to the location of juncture pause. In the original A-P forms, the final word had received major stress, whereas in the B-P forms, the penultimate word received major stress. (All excisions were made at the onset of the burst or frication of the final word of each sentence; thus the pause structure of the original version was preserved.)

For the purpose of testing, the four forms of each sentence were randomized into a fixed sequence, a recording was made, and test arrays were prepared as in Experiment 1. Administration of these materials to a new group of 26 college students revealed 93% accuracy on the control versions, 95% accuracy on the emphasized pause versions, 67% accuracy on the transposed pause versions, and 62% accuracy on the transposed stress versions. These adult subjects showed approximately equal reliance on the use of juncture pause and word stress as cues to constituent structure.

Reiterant Speech Materials.   An accurate test of children's ability to perceive the relevant prosodic cues should involve meaningless materials, since differences in meaning might confound performance on a perceptual task (see Forster, 1979, for a discussion of the role of higher level syntactic processing in performance on low-level perceptual-matching tasks). Accordingly, our perceptual test used reiterant speech versions of the A, − Article and B, − Article sentences from Experiment 1. To produce reiterant speech, a speaker is trained to say a sentence but to replace each syllable with "ma." This has the virtue of destroying utterance meaning and lexical content but preserving prosodic structure (Liberman & Prince, 1977).

Perception was assessed with a "same-different" paradigm in which the items were pairs of reiterant speech versions of the A-P and B-P test materials from Experiment 1. A female native speaker of English produced four items from each core pair of sentences, two that compared versions of the same sentence and two that compared the A and B versions. The 24 items (6 pairs × 4 items) were recorded in a fixed random order with a 3-sec isi separating the sentences in each item and a 6-sec isi between items. Adult subjects were 100% accurate in discriminating these materials.

Memory Tests.   These materials comprised a test of word-string memory and a test of memory for Corsi block sequences. The word-string memory test presented five-word strings of nonrhyming, high-frequency words (Thorndike-Lorge A and AA, 1944) at a rate of one per second. A practice string and the six test items were read aloud by the same speaker who produced the other materials for Experiment 2.

The apparatus for the Corsi block test has been described elsewhere (Kolb & Whishaw, 1985). The experimenter uses it to tap out a sequence of blocks, which the subject attempts to repeat. We followed a procedure, analogous to that used by Mann and Liberman (1984), of presenting four 2-block sequences, four 3-block sequences, four 4-block sequences, and four 5-block sequences for immediate recall. All sequences were randomly determined, and blocks were tapped at the rate of one per second.

Procedure

The sentence comprehension test and the reiterant speech discrimination test were presented to groups of children in a single experimental session, whereas the memory tests and perception tests were individually administered. The procedure for the sentence test was analogous to that in Experiment 1. For the reiterant speech test, children were told that they would be listening to a kind of "baby talk." They were given numbered response sheets on which they were to write "D" when an item contained two different "sentences" and "S" when it contained the same sentence. For the word-string recall test, subjects were told that they would be hearing five words and that, after all five had been heard, they should try to repeat them, in order. For the Corsi block test, children were instructed to watch as the experimenter touched a series of blocks, and when she stopped they were to try to touch the same blocks, in order.

RESULTS

The previous experiment had shown that children's age and reading ability are related to the ability to use prosodic cues. The second experiment reveals that poor readers and younger children can perceive prosodic cues as well as good readers and older children. However, their comprehension of spoken sentences is less sensitive to certain manipulations of prosodic structure, and this associates with a decreased memory for word strings.

Sentence Comprehension When Prosodic Structure Is Altered

The data from this test were scored in a manner analogous to that in Experiment 1. They are summarized in Figure 4.3 as a function of the mean percentage of correct responses on each version (A and B) and each of the four forms of item according to children's age and reading ability. There was a main effect of age, $F(1,36) = 16.61, p < .000$ (MSE = 28.64), but no main effect of reading ability. Here, as in Experiment 1, the "compound noun" bias is evident, with all children tending to make fewer errors on the B version, $F(1,36) = 182.96, p < .000$ (MSE = 150.01), and this interacts with reading ability, $F(1,36) = 10.06,$ $p < .003$ (MSE = 8.25), but not with age. Once again, there was no difference between the fourth-grade poor readers and their RAM controls in overall performance or in susceptibility to the various manipulations of form and version.

The main purpose of this study was to determine whether the effects of manipulated prosodic structure were a function of age and reading ability, thus the focus of the analysis was directed toward interactions involving these effects. In general, the type of manipulation had significant effects on all groups of subjects, $F(3,108) = 5.73, p < .001$ (MSE = 6.41), which were greater for the *better* readers, $F(3,108) = 6.69,$ $p < .000$ (MSE = 7.47), and the *older* children, $F(3,108) = 10.4, p < .000$ (MSE = 11.64), as can be seen in Figure 4.3. In further agreement with the suggestion that the compound noun bias might reflect poor use of prosodic cues, we found a significant three-way interaction between

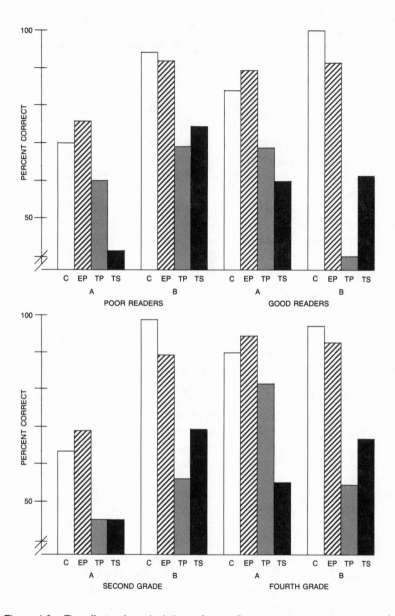

Figure 4.3. The effects of manipulations of prosodic structure on sentence comprehension. The comprehension of normal sentences (C) is compared to that in which the juncture pause is lengthened (EP), the juncture pause is transposed (TP), and the stressed words are transposed (TS), for sentences that contain a compound noun (B) and those that do not (A). The effects of reading ability appear in the top panel; those of age appear below.

version, type of manipulation, and reading ability, $F(3,108) = 5.11$, $p < .002$ (MSE = 3.37), and between version, type of manipulation, and age, $F(3,108) = 3.05$, $p < .001$ (MSE = 1.35). (There was also a significant interaction between version and type of manipulation in both analyses, $F(3,108) = 11.55$, $p < .000$ (MSE = 7.62); $F(3,48) = 3.96$, $p < .01$ (MSE = 3.19). All other interactions were nonsignificant.)

Newman-Keuls tests were conducted as a means of determining whether the poor readers' and younger children's bias toward the compound noun interpretation (i.e., the interpretation appropriate to B-version sentences) was accompanied by increased tolerance of the manipulations of prosodic structure. On the control sentences, the good readers and poor readers differed marginally on the A versions, $q_r(3,108) = 3.93$, $p < .05$, but not on the B versions. Older and younger children significantly differed on the A versions, $q_r(7,108) = 7.76$, $p < .01$, but not on the B versions. On the extended pause sentences, the poor readers made more errors than the good readers on the A versions, $q_r(4,108) = 3.93$, $p < .05$, but the difference was not significant in the B versions. A similar pattern obtained for the younger versus older children; differences were significant only for the A versions, $q_r(7,108) = 7.31$, $p < .01$. Thus we see that the compound bias was again evidenced through the greater success of poor readers and younger children on the B versions of the normal test sentences. Turning now to the manipulations that should disrupt use of prosodic cues, we predicted that, for younger children and poor readers, these disruptions would have less of an effect on the comprehension of B version sentences, where their bias leads them to adopt the correct answer. On the transposed pause sentences, the performance of both groups of subjects declined, but the poor readers made *fewer* errors than the good readers on the B − versions, $q_r(7,108) = -7.78$, $p < .01$, and they made as many errors as good readers on the A versions. Thus it is apparent that placing the pause in the incorrect place tended to be more disruptive of the performance of the good readers. Also, the fact that poor readers made fewer errors on the B version items is consistent with the suggestion that poor readers adopt a compound noun bias when they cannot make full use of prosodic cues. In the case of this manipulation, the effects of age are less clear; both older and younger children seem to be affected and the only significant difference involves the fact that younger children made more errors on the A versions $q_r(10,208) = 1.73$, $p < .01$. This result is, at least, consistent with the possibility that a bias toward the B reading is adopted by young children, but is not strongly supportive. Finally, on the transposed stress sentences, poor readers made more errors than good readers on the A versions, $q_r(2,108) = 4.75$, $p < .01$, but performed equivalently on the B versions. Younger children performed at the same level as older children on both A and B versions, offering further evidence that they are more tolerant of the disruption.

Discrimination of Prosodic Cues

Table 4.1 summarizes the results of this test in terms of the mean percentage of correct responses on each type of item according to children's age and reading ability. There is neither an effect of age nor an effect of reading ability.

An ANOVA also showed that the subjects performed comparably on both the same and different items, whether the A form or the B form occurred first. Comparison of the fourth-grade poor readers and the RAM controls revealed no effects of age or item structure. Finally, performance on this test failed to correlate with performance on either of the comprehension tests administered in Experiment 1.

Short-term Memory Tests

Responses to this test were scored according to how accurately they preserved both the identity and the order of the words/blocks in the original item. Figure 4.4 gives the mean percentage of correct responses on each test, according to children's age and reading ability.

TABLE 4.1
Reiterant Speech Discrimination
(Percentage Correct Responses)

Subject Group	"Same"		"Different"	
	A/A	B/B	A/B	B/A
Second graders: Good readers:	88.3	83.3	80.0	83.3
Second graders: Poor readers	87.0	88.9	83.3	87.0
Fourth graders: Good readers	93.0	94.5	95.8	95.8
Fourth graders: Poor readers	94.5	83.3	92.7	83.3
Second graders: Reading-ability-matched controls	90.5	88.9	92.7	88.7

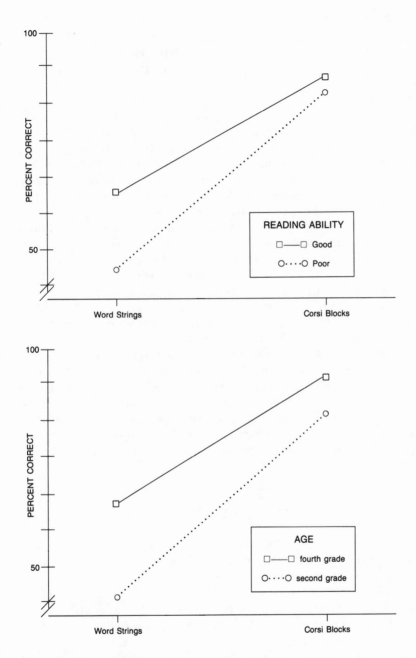

Figure 4.4. The parallel effects of reading ability and age on short-term memory performance. The effects of reading ability appear in the upper panel; those of age appear below. Each panel compares performance on the linguistic test of word string memory with that on the nonlinguistic Corsi block test of visual-spatial memory.

More errors were made, in general, by poorer readers, $F(1,39) =$ 20.84, $p < .000$ (MSE = 590.06), and younger children, $F(1,36) = 20.33$, $p < .000$ (MSE = 575.74), although the fourth-grade poor readers did not differ from the RAM controls. In general, there were fewer errors on the Corsi block test, $F(1,36) = 73.48$, $p < .000$ (MSE = 2007.89). Consistent with previous findings about the verbal memory impairments of poor readers, the poorer readers, $F(1,36) = 5.8$, $p < .021$ (MSE = 158.58), especially the older ones, $F(1,36) = 4.02$, $p < .05$ (MSE = 109.86), made more errors than the better readers on the word-string memory test, as compared to the Corsi block test. The fourth-grade poor readers and the RAM controls performed equivalently, however, on the two tests, and there was no interaction between task and age. All other interactions fell short of significance ($p > .1$).

Correlations between performance on the word-string memory test and performance on the sentence comprehension test (as measured in Experiment 1) were significant, $r(40) = .65$, $p < .001$ for the order-strict score and $r(40) = .48$, $p < .001$ for the order-free score. Correlations between word-string recall and the Noun Phrase Comprehension Test were likewise significant, $r(40) = .53$ for order strict and $r(40) = .46$ for order free. Performance on this test was also correlated with discrimination of the reiterant speech materials, $r(40) = .35$ for order strict and $r(40) = .41$, $p < .004$ for order free. When the effects of age differences between the second and fourth graders are partialed out, all of these correlations remain significant. Correlations between Corsi block recall and sentence comprehension were $r(40) = .46$ for order strict and $r(40) = .47$ for order free; these correlations become insignificant when the effects of age are partialed out. Correlations between Corsi block performance and noun phrase comprehension fell short of significance.

DISCUSSION

The results of Experiment 2 make four points. First, they indicate that poor readers and younger children perceive prosodic cues just as well as other children do. All children were equally able to discriminate the reiterant speech versions of the sentences we employed in the first experiment. Also, contrary to Scholes et al.'s (1976) speculation about the role of juncture pause perception in young children's comprehension difficulties, doubling the size of the juncture pause failed to improve the comprehension of either younger children or poor readers.

Second, although there is little indication that good and poor readers, older and younger children differed in perception of prosodic cues, there is evidence that they differ in the use of those cues. Neither the disruptions of juncture pause location nor the disruptions of word stress penalized the performance of younger children and poor readers as extensively as they penalized older children, good readers, and adults. In particular, the performance of the poor readers was most tolerant of disrupted cues in the case of the B versions of the test sentences—the sentences for which the compound noun bias yielded the correct answer. Thus we find evidence that their compound noun bias associates with a decreased reliance on prosodic cues.

Third, there is evidence that decreased reliance on prosodic cues associates with limitations on phonological coding in linguistic working memory. As other research has shown, poor readers are impaired in the ability to recall word strings (i.e., a measure of the ability to use phonological representation in working memory), yet in the present study showed effectively no impairment on the Corsi block test (i.e., a measure of visual spatial working memory). Also, all children's performance on the word-string memory test was significantly related to their performance on each of the two comprehension tests employed in Experiment 1, even when we remove the rather large differences between older and younger children from the correlation equation. Performance on the Corsi test was not related to noun phrase comprehension, and any relation to sentence comprehension became nonsignificant when the differences between older and younger children were controlled.

Fourth and finally, the data of Experiment 2 confirm and extend the maturational account of poor readers' impairments. In general, most of the similarities and differences between good and poor readers found parallels in the behavior of older versus younger children. It is interesting to note that, in the memory test, the extent of difference between good and poor readers is greatest for the word strings, whereas that between older and younger children remains the same for the word strings and the Corsi block sequences. An asymmetry of this sort suggests that, although both linguistic and nonlinguistic working memory develop with age, only the linguistic working memory system develops more slowly in poor readers. At odds with this result is the finding that the older poor readers performed at the same level as the younger RAM controls on both linguistic and nonlinguistic tests, and this conflict prevents us from concluding that language processing skills are the only realm in which poor readers are "delayed."

GENERAL DISCUSSION

We have reported the results of two experiments that confirm and extend the observation that poor readers tend to encounter phonological processing problems that lead them to misunderstand certain types of phrases and sentences. Our materials were phrases and sentences that exploited the prosodic cues of pitch, pause, and stress, and they have shown us that poor readers do not use prosodic cues as effectively as good readers do. These children tend to be less able to understand spoken utterances when grammatical structure is disambiguated by nuances of pitch, stress, and pause, not because they fail to perceive those cues so much as because they fail to hold them in working memory. We cannot attribute the poor readers' comprehension errors to a misperception of prosodic cues, because they neither profit from enhanced cues nor fail to discriminate similar cues in nonsense materials. Instead, we find a significant correlation between comprehension accuracy and the ability to hold spoken word strings in working memory. Here, as in other cases, the comprehension problems of the poor readers may be due to a processing limitation that, by compromising phonological working memory capacity, prevents the child from fully recovering the structure of spoken language (see Shankweiler & Crain, 1986, for further discussion).

Our results, and other observations that have been reported in the literature, give us little reason to conclude that poor readers possess an insufficient grammatical knowledge of syntax. Here, as in other experiments (Mann et al., 1984; Smith, 1987; Smith et al., 1987), although poor readers are biased toward certain interpretations, their bias reflects processing limitations (i.e., poor use of cues that mark syntactic structure) rather than insufficient knowledge of sentence structure, as such. Others have speculated that the compound noun bias seen among the poor readers and younger children in our study might reflect poor knowledge of the double object construction. The study of Fletcher et al. (1981) is a case in point; it used sentences like those of Experiment 1 to test the possibility that measures of syntactic skill contribute differentially to reading achievement at different ages. The results indicated significant differences in the compound noun bias of good and poor readers in the fifth grade that were not present among third graders or kindergarten children who became good and poor readers in the second grade. However, interpretation is confounded by three problems inherent in the test battery: the failure to consider the importance of prosodic cues, the exclusive use of a small set of sentences, and the use of a single syntactic structure. We avoided these confounding factors by using an expanded set of sentences that stressed the use of prosodic cues, and we discovered significant differences between good and poor readers at two different ages, second and fourth grade, which held for both sentences and noun phrases that, although shorter and less embedded than the sentences, stress the use of prosodic cues, A compound noun bias was evident for the sentences, but not for the noun phrases, and we further found some evidence that the compound noun bias associates with poor use of prosodic cues. This pattern of results, together with the other evidence that all of our materials involved syntactic structures that are within the grasp of young children and poor readers, makes us question whether a lack of syntactic knowledge explains the compound noun bias in this and other studies.

Both of our experiments were designed not only to elucidate the role of phonological processing problems in the sentence comprehension of poor readers, but also to test one explanation of these problems: a maturational delay in language development. It is consistent with a maturational lag account that we found parallel effects of age and reading ability throughout all phases of our study. We further discovered that the fourth-grade poor readers in our sample were indistinguishable from second-grade average readers. These groups were indistinguishable both in the level of their performance and in their susceptibility to various manipulations of our test materials. We do not view it likely that the resemblance between poor readers and slightly younger children is a consequence of similar reading vocabularies and similar experiences with written material, for the results that we have obtained involved the use of spoken language materials that exploit prosodic cues that are not systematically marked in written language. This fact leads us to interpret the resemblance between poor readers and slightly younger children as evidence that they occupy more or less the same position on some developmental continuum of spoken language processing skill.

Before leaving this topic, we would like to note the possibility that many of the poor readers who are delayed in the acquisition of phonological skills may never catch up with their nondelayed peers. Indeed, several studies are finding that many of the special characteristics of disabled readers in the elementary school years still hold in adolescence (Holmes & McKeever, 1979; McKeever & Van Deventer, 1975) and beyond (Jackson & McClelland, 1979; Read & Ruyter, 1985; Russell, 1982; Scarborough, 1984). This evidence prompts us to speculate that delays in early language development might associate with inferior language skills at maturity, perhaps because they interact with other biological factors to produce a premature plateau in the normal maturational sequence. It is hoped that future projects will address this point.

SOME PRACTICAL APPLICATIONS

Certainly it is important to discern the differences between good and poor readers, and to clarify their bases; it is equally important to ask what practical advantages this knowledge can offer. Therefore, in concluding, we would like to note just a few practical implications of this type of research. One implication concerns the common classroom observation that poor readers do not follow instructions as well as other children do. This problem is entirely to be expected from the fact that poor readers have difficulty with sentences that are unusually long, especially those that contain complex embedded relative clauses (as discussed in Mann et al., 1984) and those that stress the use of prosodic cues. It might be a good idea to avoid such structures, especially when giving instructions to poor readers.

Perhaps the most interesting implication of sentence comprehension tests like those in this and other studies concerns their potential for screening preschool-aged children for future reading problems. Unlike most of the phonological tests that have been considered in our previous research (see, for example, Mann, 1984b; Mann & Liberman, 1984), sentence comprehension tests lend themselves to group testing. In progress is a study in which we are examining kindergarten performance on a variety of linguistic and nonlinguistic measures; these include an invented spelling test (Mann et al., 1987) and several other group tests of phonological awareness, and the group sentence comprehension test that was used in Experiment 1. Performance on this test battery is now being related to children's first-grade reading ability. While it is too early to report a complete analysis of the results, there are indications that sentence comprehension can be a sensitive predictor of future reading ability, especially when combined with the tests of phonological awareness.

REFERENCES

Backman, J.E., Mamen, M., & Ferguson, H.B. (1984). Reading level design: Conceptual and methodological issues in reading research. *Psychological Bulletin, 96,* 560–568.

Brady, S., Mann, V.A., & Schmidt, R. (1987). Errors in short-term memory for good and poor readers. *Memory and Cognition, 15,* 444–453.

Brady, S., Shankweiler, D., & Mann, V. (1983). Speech perception and memory coding in relation to reading ability. *Journal of Experimental Child Psychology, 35,* 345–367.

Bryant, P., & Goswami, U. (1986). Strengths and weaknesses of the reading level design: A comment on Backman, Mamen and Ferguson. *Psychological Bulletin, 100,* 101–103.

Fischer, F.W., Liberman, I.Y., & Shankweiler, D. (1977). Reading reversals and developmental dyslexia: A further study. *Cortex, 14,* 496–510.

Fletcher, J.M., Satz, P., & Scholes, R. (1981). Developmental changes in the linguistic performance correlates of reading achievements. *Brain and Language, 13,* 78–90.

Forster, K.I. (1979). Levels of processing and the structure of the language processor. In W.E. Cooper & W.C.T. Walker (Eds.), *Sentence processing: Psycholinguistic studies presented to Merrill Garrett* (pp. 27–86). Hillsdale, NJ: Erlbaum.

Gleitman, L., & Wanner, E. (1982). Language acquisition: The state of the art. In L. Gleitman & E. Wanner (Eds.), *Language acquisition: The state of the art* (pp. 3–48). Cambridge, England: Cambridge University Press.

Grosjean, F., Grosjean, L., & Lane, H. (1979). The patterns of silence: Performance structures in sentence production. *Cognitive Psychology, 11,* 58–81.

Hamburger, H., & Crain, S. (1984). Acquisition of cognitive compiling. *Cognition, 17,* 85–136.

Holmes, D.R., & McKeever, W.F. (1979). Material specific serial memory deficit in adolescent dyslexics. *Cortex, 15,* 51–62.

Jackson, M., & McClelland, J.L. (1979). Processing determinants of reading speed. *Journal of Experimental Psychology: General, 108,* 151–181.

Jorm, A.F. (1979). The cognitive and neurological basis of developmental dyslexia: A theoretical framework and review. *Cognition, 7,* 19–33.

Jorm, A.F. (1983). Specific reading retardation and working memory: A review. *British Journal of Psychology, 74,* 311–342.

Jorm, A.F., & Share, D.L. (1983). Phonological recoding and reading acquisition. *Applied Psycholinguistics, 4,* 103–147.

Kolb, B., & Whishaw, I.Q. (1985). *Fundamentals of human neuropsychology.* New York: W.H. Freeman.

Liberman, I.Y. (1983). A language-oriented view of reading and its disabilities. In H. Myklebust (Ed.), *Progress in learning disabilities: Volume 5* (pp. 81–101). New York: Grune & Stratton.

Liberman, I.Y., & Mann, V.A. (1980). Should reading remediation vary with the sex of the child? In A. Ansara, N. Geschwind, A. Galaburda, N. Albert, & N. Gartrell (Eds.), *Sex differences in dyslexia* (pp. 151–167). Towson, MD: The Orton Dyslexia Society.

Liberman, I.Y., Mann, V.A., Shankweiler, D., & Werfelman, M. (1982). Children's memory for recurring linguistic and non-linguistic material in relation to reading ability. *Cortex, 18,* 367–375.

Liberman, M., & Prince, A. (1977). On stress and linguistic rhythm. *Linguistic Inquiry, 8,* 249–336.

Mann, V.A. (1984a). Reading skill and language skill. *Developmental Review, 4,* 1–15.

Mann, V.A. (1984b). Longitudinal prediction and prevention of early reading disability. *Annals of Dyslexia, 34,* 117–136.

Mann, V.A. (1986). Why some children encounter reading problems: The contribution of difficulties with language processing and phonological sophistication to early reading difficulty. In J.K. Torgesen & B.Y. Wong (Eds.), *Learning disabilities: Some new perspectives* (pp. 133–159). New York: Academic Press.

Mann, V.A, & Liberman, I.Y. (1984). Phonological awareness and verbal short-term memory. *Journal of Learning Disabilities, 17,* 592–599.

Mann, V.A., Liberman, I.Y., & Shankweiler, D. (1980). Children's memory for sentences and words in relation to reading ability. *Memory and Cognition, 8,* 329–335.

Mann, V.A., Shankweiler, D., & Smith, S. (1984). The association between comprehension of spoken sentences and early reading ability: The role of phonetic representation. *Journal of Child Language, 11,* 627–643.

Mann, V.A., Tobin, P., & Wilson, R. (1987). Measuring phonological awareness through the invented spellings of kindergarten children. *Merrill-Palmer Quarterly, 33,* 364–392.

Matthei, E.M. (1982). The acquisition of prenominal modifier sequences. *Cognition, 11,* 301–332.

McKeever, W.F., & Van Deventer, A.D. (1975). Dyslexic adolescents: Evidence of impaired visual and auditory language processing associated with normal lateralization and visual responsivity. *Cortex, 11,* 361–378.

Pinker, S. (1984). *Language learnability and language development.* Cambridge, MA: Harvard University Press.

Rayner, K. (1985). Do faulty eye movements cause dyslexia? *Developmental Neuropsychology, 1,* 3–15.

Read, C., & Ruyter, L. (1985). Reading and spelling skills in adults of low literacy. *Reading and Special Education, 6,* 8–17.

Robinson, M.E., & Schwartz, L.B. (1973). Visuo-motor skills and reading ability: A longitudinal study. *Developmental Medicine and Child Neurology, 15,* 280–286.

Russell, G., (1982). Impairment of phonetic reading in dyslexia and its persistence beyond childhood—Research note. *Journal of Child Psychology and Child Psychiatry, 23,* 459–475.

Scarborough, H.S. (1984). Continuity between childhood dyslexia and adult reading. *British Journal of Psychology, 75,* 329–348.

Scholes, R.J., Tanis, D.C., & Turner, A. (1976). Syntactic and strategic aspects of the comprehension of indirect and direct constructions by children. *Language and Speech, 19,* 212–223.

Shankweiler, D., & Crain, S. (1986). Language mechanisms and reading disorder: A modular approach. *Cognition, 24,* 139–168.

Shankweiler, D., & Liberman, I.Y. (1976). Exploring the relations between reading and speech. In R.M. Knights & D.K. Bakker (Eds.), *Neuropsychology of learning disorders: Theoretical approaches* (pp. 293–317). Austin, TX: PRO-ED.

Shankweiler, D., Smith, S., & Mann, V.A. (1984). Repetition and comprehension of spoken sentences by reading-disabled children. *Brain and Language, 23,* 241–257.

Simner, M.L. (1982). Printing errors in kindergarten and the prediction of academic performance. *Journal of Learning Disabilities, 15,* 155–159.

Smith, S. (1987). *Syntactic comprehension in reading-disabled children.* Unpublished doctoral dissertation, University of Connecticut, Storrs.

Smith, S.T., Mann, V.A., & Shankweiler, D. (1986). Spoken sentence comprehension by good and poor readers: A study with the Token test. *Cortex, 22,* 627–632.

Smith, S.T., Mann, V.A., & Shankweiler, D. (1987). Token test performance by good and poor readers. *Cortex, 24,* 435–447.

Stanovich, K.E. (1985). Explaining the variance in reading ability in terms of pyschological processes: What have we learned? *Annals of Dyslexia, 35,* 67–96.

Stanovich, K.E. (1988). Explaining the differences between the dyslexic and the garden-variety poor reader: The phonological-core variable-difference model. *Journal of Learning Disabilities, 21,* 590–604.

Stanovich, K.E., Cunningham, A.E., & Freeman, D.J. (1984). Intelligence, cognitive skills and early reading progress. *Reading Research Quarterly, 14,* 279–303.

Stanovich, K.E., Nathan, R.G., & Vala-Rossi, M. (in press). Developmental changes in the cognitive correlates of reading ability and the developmental lag hypothesis. *Reading Research Quarterly.*

Streeter, L.A. (1978). Acoustic determinants of phrase boundary perception. *Journal of the Acoustical Society of America, 64,* 1582–1592.

Vellutino, F.R. (1979). *Dyslexia: Theory and research.* Cambridge, MA: MIT Press.

Wagner, R.K., & Torgesen, J.K. (1987). The nature of phonological processing and its causal role in the acquisition of reading skills. *Psychological Bulletin, 101,* 192–212.

Woodcock, R.W. (1973). *Woodcock reading mastery tests.* Circle Pines, MN: American Guidance Service.

5. Cognitive Deficits in Reading Disability and Attention Deficit Disorder

REBECCA H. FELTON AND FRANK B. WOOD

Specific reading disability (RD) and attention deficit disorder (ADD) often coexist. On the one hand, children referred for academic problems frequently have a substantially greater than normal incidence of significant attentional problems (Holobrow & Berry, 1986; Levine, Busch, & Aufsuser, 1982; Shaywitz, 1986). On the other hand, children in samples chosen for primary attentional problems commonly have academic problems—more so than do children with most other psychiatric diagnoses (Barnes & Forness, 1982; Cantwell & Satterfield, 1978; Lambert & Sandoval, 1980). Nonetheless, despite the empirical fact of greater-than-chance overlap between RD and ADD, there is no clear theoretical consensus about the nature of the disorders in isolation, still less about their overlap.

A major issue is about the primacy of one disorder in cases in which the disorders coexist. Douglas and Peters (1979) proposed the following distinction: Children with attention deficit disorder (ADD) have constitutional impairments in attentional mechanisms, and their learning problems are secondary; on the other hand, children with learning disabilities (LD) have basic processing problems, and their

This research was supported by PHS Grant NS 19413 to the University of North Carolina–Greensboro, subcontract to Bowman Gray School of Medicine PHS Grant No. P01HD21887-01 to Bowman Gray School of Medicine.

failure experiences in school lead to frustration and secondary attentional problems. Several reviews have supported this distinction,
especially those concluding that attentional problems constitute a
secondary overlay rather than a primary cause of specific reading
disabilities (Fleisher, Soodak, & Jelin, 1984; Koppell, 1979; Vellutino
& Scanlon, 1982).

In a broader approach, Kinsbourne and Caplan (1979) suggest
that each disorder is primary in its own sphere (processing power
deficits in RD, maldistribution of attention in ADD), but that either
can cause significant school problems. Indeed, Kinsbourne and Caplan
believe that a major clinical/diagnostic issue for individual children
is precisely the question of primacy—an issue of practical importance
since the diagnosis of attentional primacy may lead to effective treatment with stimulant medication in some cases, whereas the diagnosis
of a primary basic processing disorder conveys no expectation of direct
benefit from stimulants.

A more cognitive and neuropsychological analysis is provided by
Dykman and colleagues (Ackerman, Anhalt, Dykman, & Holcomb, 1986;
Ackerman & Dykman, 1982; Ackerman, Dykman, & Oglesby, 1983;
Dykman, Ackerman, Holcomb, & Bondreau, 1983). Children with ADD
are viewed as having deficits in *sustained* attention, attributable to fron-
tal and limbic dysfunction. In contrast, children with RD are thought
to have problems in *selective* attention, attributable to temporal lobe
dysfunction. Although the attentional problems of children with RD
may be similar in some respects to those of children with ADD, in
children with RD these difficulties will surface only in situations that
stress their already impaired information processing (selective attention) capabilities (Dykman, Ackerman, & Holcomb, 1985).

From a different perspective, Kinsbourne (1982) maintained that
the essence of selective attention is preparation or adoption of the
correct mental set. Selective attention problems may then interact with
or even cause cognitive processing problems, as when children with
RD have difficulty with rapid automatized naming because of failure
to maintain the proper verbal set (i.e., attend selectively to names of
items rather than to other attributes). See, however, Krupski's (1986)
evidence that both LD and ADD children tend to show task- or situation-
specific (not generalized) deficits in sustained attention, involving
embedded rather than distal distractors. Given such specificity, Krupski
contends, it is not useful to invoke a generalized attentional disorder:
Specific deficits—giving rise to the specific tasks or situations eliciting
the impaired attention—should instead be sought.

The theoretical questions often lead to research designs intended
to distinguish between ADD and RD children on a variety of cognitive
measures. Thus, in a study that compared three clinical groups

(NoRD/ADD, RD/NoADD, RD/ADD) to controls, Dykman et al. (1985) found no group differences on measures of automaticity (speed of picture naming and writing letters), and all three clinical groups were significantly impaired on arithmetic in comparison to controls. Only on an acoustic-semantic memory task were there significant differences between clinical groups, with the RD subjects performing more poorly on the phonological component of the task. Bohline (1985) compared ADD with NoADD groups in a heterogeneous group of students referred for academic problems and found no significant differences on any subtests of the Woodcock-Johnson Test of Cognitive Abilities. Halperin, Gittelman, Klein, and Rudel (1984) administered a variety of intellectual and neuropsychological tests to children classified as mixed (ADD/RD) or pure (ADD/NoRD), and concluded that there were no clear differences between ADD children with and without reading difficulties.

More positive results (Halperin et al., 1984; Lahey, Stempniak, Robinson, & Tyroler, 1978) in the domain of general deportment and classroom behavior nevertheless continue to keep alive the notion that ADD and RD are independent factors that can exist in isolation.

The extant studies use such a variety of designs and definitions of subjects that it is not yet possible to explain them all by a single theoretical solution. In our view, what is therefore required is a series of replicated studies with a variety of converging operations, so that a more comprehensive and consistent theoretical picture can be assembled from the now divergent and sometimes discrepant data. Obviously, any such program must simultaneously study both ADD and RD, in as broad a population as possible.

Our research has concentrated on separating the effects of attention deficit disorder and reading disability on a broad spectrum of cognitive processes. In this chapter, we present three studies that address these issues in different ways—a cross-sectional study of school-referred children, a test-retest study of children classified as specific subtypes of RD, and a study of a large, randomly selected group of first graders. Methodologically we are concerned with examining several different sources of variance, for example, differences in intelligence, that present possible confounds in studies of specific cognitive skills. This naturally leads to the use of multivariate statistical procedures in which such factors as age and IQ are considered along with RD and ADD as having a role in the prediction of specific cognitive test performance. Such a use of standard tests of basic verbal and nonverbal ability as control measures is one good approach to the differential deficit issue, which is close to the heart of the theoretical questions at stake. Analyses that measure and control for general verbal and nonverbal ability can thus separate general intellectual deficit from more specific cognitive deficits. (See Chapman & Chapman, 1973, for one particularly cogent methodological discussion of this problem.)

STUDY 1

Study 1 (Felton, Wood, Brown, Campbell, & Harter, 1987) investigated verbal memory and naming deficits in reading disabled and control children who were characterized according to the presence or absence of attention deficit disorder. Subjects with reading disabilities (RD) were 45 children (41 males and 4 females, ages 8 to 12) who had been diagnosed as learning disabled by North Carolina state guidelines (i.e., a discrepancy of at least 1 ½ years between expected and actual reading level). NoRD subjects were 53 children (41 males and 12 females, ages 8 to 12) who were identified by school personnel as having at least average ability in reading and at least average intelligence as measured by group intelligence tests. Initial subject selection and group assignment were carried out without regard to the presence or absence of attention deficit disorder.

Assessment instruments were selected to reflect certain aspects of word retrieval, rapid automatized naming, verbal memory, and verbal fluency that have been implicated in reading disability. Measures included the Peabody Picture Vocabulary Test–Revised (PPVT-R) (Dunn & Dunn, 1981), the Boder Test of Reading/Spelling Patterns (Boder & Jarrico, 1982), the Boston Naming Test (Kaplan, Goodglass, & Weintraub, 1982), the Rapid Automatized Naming Tests (digits, colors, letters, and objects), the Verbal Fluency Test (semantic and linguistic) (Benton & Hamsher, 1976; Lezak, 1983), the Rey Auditory Verbal Learning Test (Rey, 1964; Taylor, 1959), and the Prose Recall— The Cowboy Story (immediate and delayed recall) (Talland, 1965).

In addition, the Attention Deficit Disorder (ADD) portion of the Diagnostic Interview for Children and Adolescents (DICA) by Herjanic (1983) was administered to a parent or guardian of each subject. The DICA is a structured interview intended to standardize and operationalize Diagnostic and Statistical Manual of Mental Disorders (3rd ed.) diagnoses. With DICA criteria for ADD, each child was classified as ADD or NoADD. Although the DICA interview data allowed for the diagnosis of ADD with and without hyperactivity, so few of the subjects (only 5 RD and 1 NoRD) were ADD without hyperactivity that the analysis was carried out without regard to this distinction.

The main effects of ADD and RD and the interaction of ADD and RD were tested in a general linear model that included age and PPVT-R standard score as covariates. Data from the neuropsychological measures were entered as dependent variables. A multivariate analysis was conducted on the entire model, followed by separate univariate analyses on each of the dependent measures.

The overall multivariate analysis of covariance showed significant main effects for reading disability, attention deficit disorder, age, and PPVT-R with no interaction between ADD and RD. Univariate tests of the main effects for each dependent variable are presented in Table 5.1 and can be summarized as follows: The free recall on the distractor trial of the Rey Auditory Verbal Learning Test (RAVLT) as well as the immediate and delayed Prose Recall were unrelated either to ADD or RD; confrontation naming on the Boston Naming Test as well as rapid automatized naming of digits, letters, colors, and objects were all significant for the RD effect only; free recalls on the first and fifth trials and the postdistractional trial of the RAVLT were significant for the ADD main effect only; and both linguistic and semantic types of verbal fluency were significant for both the RD and ADD main effects.

TABLE 5.1

Test Performance as a Function of Absence (NoADD) or Presence (ADD) of Attention Deficit Disorder and Absence (NoRD) or Presence (RD) of Reading Disability, in the Full Sample ($N = 98$), Reported as Mean (Standard Deviation)

Variable	NoRD		RD	
	NoAdd	ADD	NoADD	ADD
Boston Naming Test	44.82(5.97)#	43.00(5.98)	35.84(7.15)	35.77(6.51)
Rapid Naming of Digits	24.20(5.01)#	27.31(9.35)	31.21(7.66)	35.85(11.77)
Rapid Naming of Letters	23.85(4.20)#	26.85(5.46)	35.32(11.63)	38.77(14.40)
Rapid Naming of Colors	41.70(7.82)#	43.00(8.52)	50.00(11.92)	54.08(19.47)
Rapid Naming of Objects	47.70(8.83)#	54.23(16.68)	75.95(24.46)	65.73(17.64)
Linguistic Fluency	30.45(9.14)#*	24.00(4.51)	21.63(6.99)	21.12(6.24)
Semantic Fluency	35.40(7.58)#*	30.00(6.23)	29.63(7.48)	27.08(5.67)
RAVLT Trial 1	6.25(1.61)*	5.54(1.61)	5.89(1.41)	4.77(1.11)
RAVLT Trial 5	12.12(1.60)*	11.00(2.86)	12.11(2.45)	10.85(2.27)
RAVLT Distractor Trial	5.35(1.42)	4.85(1.68)	5.21(1.75)	4.92(1.87)
RAVLT Postdistractor Trial	10.77(1.93)*	9.62(3.25)	10.89(2.16)	8.92(2.33)
Prose Recall, Immediate	11.73(4.43)	8.54(5.27)	10.00(4.91)	11.04(4.58)
Prose Recall, Delayed	11.00(4.47)	9.15(5.21)	8.84(5.20)	9.81(4.63)

Note. 1. In the univariate analyses with PPVT-R and age as covariates, # indicates a main effect for RD at $p < .01$; *a main effect for ADD at $p < .01$. See text for experiment-wise results.
2. RAVLT = Rey Auditory Verbal Learning Test.
3. From "Separate Verbal Memory and Naming Deficits in Attention Deficit Disorder and Reading Disability" by R.H. Felton, F.B. Wood, I.S. Brown, & S.K. Campbell, 1987, Brain and Language, 31, p. 180. Copyright 1987 by Academic Press. Reprinted by permission.

These results indicate that for this sample of children the effects of ADD and RD were on separate and distinct sets of cognitive tests with only partial overlap. Deficits in rote verbal learning and memory occurred as a function of ADD rather than RD, while deficits in word retrieval and rapid naming were specific to RD. Our interpretation was that the naming deficit in RD children was limited to those aspects of naming in which an association to an externally provided cue was required (i.e., cues provided by visual stimuli on the Boston and the Rapid Automatized Naming tests or by the categories in the verbal fluency tests). When the task did not require such associations, as on the verbal learning tests (RAVLT), no RD deficit was observed.

STUDY 2

Study 2 investigated cognitive deficits associated with subtypes of reading disabilities by evaluating naming and word retrieval skills in children classified according to subtype of reading disability as well as to the presence or absence of attention deficit disorder. The stability of the subtype classifications was also studied by test-retest comparisons of a subset of RD children (with and without ADD). The subjects for this study were the same 45 children with RD reported in Study 1.

Method

As described in Study 1, subjects were classified as RD on the basis of school testing and as ADD or NoADD based on the DICA scores, resulting in the following groups: RD/NoADD and RD/ADD. A subset of the test battery described in Study 1 was utilized for this investigation, that is, the Boston Naming Test (BNT), the Rapid Automatized Naming Tests (RAN letter, object, digit, and color), the PPVT-R, and the Boder Test of Reading/Spelling Patterns.

Following the procedures outlined by Boder and Jarrico (1982), each RD subject was classified as to reading subtype (i.e., normal, nonspecific, dysphonetic, dyseidetic, or mixed). Each child's test battery was independently scored by two examiners and, when differences in scoring occurred (on the determination of good phonetic equivalents), a consensus was reached (Kappa = .6146). Thus, each RD subject was classified as to the presence or absence of ADD and Boder subtype. Because of the small numbers of subjects in each subtype, subjects in the dysphonetic ($n = 16$) and mixed dysphonetic-dyseidetic ($n = 13$) groups were combined into a language disability group and compared to subjects in the dyseidetic ($n = 5$) and nonspecific reading retardation ($n = 10$) groups (nonlanguage disability group). One RD subject was classified as a normally achieving reader on the Boder and was not included in this analysis.

According to Boder and Jarrico (1982), subjects in the dyseidetic and nonspecific groups have intact language processing skills and would, therefore, be expected to demonstrate at least average ability on the naming and word retrieval tasks. In contrast, it would be expected that some of the dysphonetic and mixed subtype subjects would demonstrate impairments on these language tasks. To evaluate possible subtype differences within the RD group on naming and word retrieval, we entered data from the rapid naming and word retrieval tasks as dependent variables in an analysis of covariance. The main effects of language disability (dysphonetic and mixed subtypes) and nonlanguage disability (nonspecific and dyseidetic subtypes) were tested with age and PPVT-R as covariates.

Results

The Boder classifications, at the initial evaluation, for the RD subjects as well as the distribution of ADD among the subtypes, are presented in Table 5.2. Of greatest importance for the purposes of this paper is the fact that ADD was not uniformly distributed across the Boder subtypes. The majority of subjects in the nonspecific, dyseidetic, and mixed subtypes were classified as ADD (80%, 80%, and 69%, respectively). In contrast, only 31% of the dysphonetic subjects were classified as ADD.

TABLE 5.2
Boder Subtype and ADD Classifications for RD Sample of $N = 45$

Subtype	ADD ($n = 26$) n	NoADD ($n = 19$) n	Total n (%)
Normal	—	1	1 (2)
Nonspecific	8	2	10 (22)
Dyseidetic	4	1	5 (11)
Dysphonetic	5	11	16 (36)
Mixed	9	4	13 (29)

Note. ADD = attention deficit disorder; RD = reading disability.

The results of the analysis of covariance testing for main effects of nonlanguage disability and language disability indicated no significant differences between subtypes on any of the naming measures. That is, within the RD sample, subjects classified as dyseidetic and nonspecific (nonlanguage disability) were as impaired, as a group, as subjects classified as dysphonetic and mixed (language disability), on the measures of naming and word retrieval (see Table 5.3). Although no statistically significant differences were found between groups when the subtypes were collapsed in this manner, analysis of the performance of individual subjects on the various naming measures indicated important differences between RD subtypes (e.g., in the number of subjects with deficits on a particular measure as well as the degree of the deficit). Some of these differences and possible interactions with attentional deficits are discussed below.

To evaluate the stability of the subtype classifications over time, we contacted the male subjects with RD for a follow-up evaluation between 13 and 24 ($X = 19$) months after the initial testing. Of the original 41 male RD subjects, 27 were available for the retest. Seventeen of these boys had been classified as ADD (13 with hyperactivity and 4 without hyperactivity) in the initial evaluation. These subjects were readministered the Boder by an examiner blind to the results of the first evaluation, and they were then classified into the appropriate Boder subtype. The results of the initial and follow-up subtype classifications were compared for changes over time in relation to specific subtypes and to ADD.

The 27 subjects with RD who were retested on the Boder were between 10 and 14 years of age (mean = 12.63) at retest and earned

TABLE 5.3
Test Performance as a Function of Subtype Classification
(Language or Nonlanguage Disability) in the RD Sample

Variable	Language ($n = 29$) (dysphonetic and mixed)		Nonlanguage ($n = 15$) (dyseidetic and nonspecific)	
	M	SD	M	SD
Boston Naming Test	13.2	(3.1)	13.4	(2.7)
RAN–digits	33.4	(9.9)	35.1	(11.8)
RAN–colors	50.4	(14.0)	56.4	(21.2)
RAN–objects	67.1	(20.8)	74.5	(21.9)
RAN–letters	38.7	(14.9)	35.2	(9.8)

Note. RAN = Rapid Automatized Naming Test; RD = reading disability.

reading quotients between 59 and 109 (mean = 72.96). Test-retest results indicated that 16 of the 27 subjects with RD (59%) changed Boder subtypes from the first to the second testing. Changes occurred within each subtype classification with 50% of the nonspecific, 66% of the dyseidetic, 50% of the dysphonetic, and 70% of the mixed subtype subjects changing classifications. Specific changes for subjects within each subtype are presented in Table 5.4. Of the 16 subjects who were classified differently from first to second evaluation, 13 (81%) were ADD.

An analysis of the test-retest changes for individual subjects suggested an explanation for some, but not all, of the changes. For example, four of the subjects classified as mixed subtype at the first testing were unclassifiable at the second testing due to improvement in their ability to apply phonics to spelling, with no comparable improvement in reading ability. This finding is consistent with the impact of particular teaching methods. More difficult to understand is the example of the subject who changed from dyseidetic to dysphonetic subtype due to a decrease in the ability to apply phonetic decoding to spelling. Given the high number of ADD children who changed subtype,

TABLE 5.4
Changes in Subtype Classifications from Test 1 to Test 2 for RD Sample of $n = 27$

Test 1 Subtype	n	Test 2 Subtype	n	Number / % Change
Nonspecific	4	Nonspecific	2	
		Dysphonetic	1	2 / 50%
		Undetermined	1	
Dyseidetic	3	Dyseidetic	1	
		Dysphonetic	1	2 / 66%
		Unclassified	1	
Dysphonetic	10	Dysphonetic	5	
		Mixed	2	
		Dyseidetic	1	5 / 50%
		Undetermined	1	
		Normal	1	
Mixed	10	Mixed	3	
		Dysphonetic	2	7 / 70%
		Dyseidetic	1	
		Unclassified	4	
	27		27	16 / 59%

Note. RD = reading disability.

it is at least plausible that some of the changes from test to test were due to attentional factors.

Discussion

As this study clearly indicates, at least one subtyping scheme (Boder's) may be strongly confounded with ADD. Even more importantly, the stability of subtype assignment over time may be, in part, dependent on whether the subject is ADD: If he or she is, then there is a strong likelihood that subtype membership will change on later retest. In this case, ADD might be considered as a condition that, if present, diminishes the long-term reliability of cognitive test measures. That would be consistent with the clinical phenomenology of unpredictable behavior in ADD, and it would offer some clarification on the issue of generalized attentional disorder: It is the very nature, by definition, of generalized attentional disorder that it will not show up consistently in all tasks and situations, but instead inconsistently and unpredictably in a variety of situations.

Although the presence of attentional problems does not appear to be sufficient basis for reading disability (as evidenced by subjects with ADD/NoRD), these data suggest that ADD may interact with the type and degree of cognitive deficit to produce reading disabilities. Within the RD sample, the subjects who were the least impaired on measures of reading (nonspecifics) as well as those who were the most severely impaired (mixed and dyseidetics) had high incidences of ADD. It is conceivable that children with mild cognitive deficits (e.g., naming or other linguistic deficits) may function adequately in reading given adequate attentional skills. However, the additional cognitive burden of an attentional problem could be sufficient to produce a reading disability. This reading problem could be relatively mild, as in the case of the nonspecific subtype, and the cognitive deficits associated with it could be difficult to ascertain unless very sensitive measures were used (e.g., rapid automatized naming). In this study, only 2 of the 10 nonspecific subjects were within normal limits on all of the RAN tests.

Conversely, it is likely that severe and pervasive cognitive deficits in areas vital to reading, coupled with attentional problems, would produce relatively intractable reading disabilities. Based on the Boder test results, the mixed subtype subjects were very impaired both in sight word acquisition and in elementary decoding skills. In addition, there were no subjects in the mixed subtype who were within the normal range on all of the RAN tests and many had extremely long latencies, particularly on the letter naming test. These results suggest that mixed subtype subjects have a combination of deficits in phonological and naming skills that may be exacerbated by attentional problems.

The dyseidetic subjects (described by Boder as having basic deficits in visual-perceptual processes with intact language skills) in this study were also significantly impaired on the rapid and confrontation naming tasks in comparison to controls. None of the dyseidetic subjects were within the normal range on all of the RAN tests. This suggests that dyseidetic readers may have mastered basic decoding skills (as evidenced by their reliance on decoding in reading and spelling), yet have significant deficits in word retrieval and rapid naming that may impair the acquisition of sight words and the development of the automaticity necessary for fluent reading. Attentional problems may serve to exacerbate such deficits (cf. Ackerman & Dykman, 1982).

In this study, dysphonetic readers had a relatively low incidence of ADD and may represent a group of poor readers with severe phonological processing problems sufficient to produce reading problems whether or not attentional problems are present. Interestingly, a subject-by-subject analysis of the RAN data revealed that a third of the dysphonetic subjects performed within the normal range on these tasks. These results concur with research by Blachman (1983) indicating that naming deficits and phonological deficits contribute separately but significantly to reading disabilities.

In summary, we corroborate other research (Liberman, 1983; Hooper & Hynd, 1985; Olson, 1985; Van den Bos, 1984; Vellutino, 1983) that challenges the Boder distinction between linguistic and visuospatial subtypes. Clearly, when sensitive tests of linguistic processing are used, the predicted between-subtype differences are not found. More importantly, we find the subtypes to be confounded by ADD, and we find ADD-confounded subtypes to be unstable over time. Although these results must be considered preliminary due to the small sample size and the limited number of cognitive skills tested, they do point to the importance of assessing attention in studies of reading disability and its putative subtypes.

STUDY 3

In order to address the methodological limitations of Study 1 (i.e., small sample size, limited number of cognitive variables, and school-referred sample), in Study 3 we investigated a wide variety of cognitive skills in a large sample of randomly selected school children who were characterized according to evidence of attentional deficits and beginning reading ability. This study is part of a project funded

by the National Institute of Child Health and Human Development
on neurobehavioral definition and subtyping of dyslexia.

Method

Subjects.   A sample of 800 children randomly selected from the entire
population ($N = 3,011$) of first graders in the Winston-Salem/Forsyth
County school system was invited to participate in this study in the
fall of the 1986–87 school year. Permission to participate in the study
was obtained from the parents of 485 children, 269 males and 216
females, who ranged in age from 6 to 8 ($\bar{X} = 7.11$). One hundred and
sixty-six (34.7%) of the study participants were minority students
compared to a minority population of 39.7% of the total first grade.

Assessment Instruments

1. Tests of reading:

   Woodcock-Johnson Psycho-Educational Battery–Reading Cluster
(WJPB) (Woodcock & Johnson, 1977). The reading cluster of the
Woodcock (WJPB) measures letter-word identification, word attack,
and passage comprehension.

   Decoding Skills Test (Richardson & DeBenedetto, 1985). The
Decoding Skills Test (DST), developed as a research tool for use in
studies of dyslexia, contains three subtests: basal word recognition,
phonic decoding, and oral reading.

2. Tests of cognitive skills, including:
   Tests of specific language functions:
   Boston Naming Test (BNT)
   Rapid Automatized Naming (RAN)
   Auditory-Verbal Learning Test (RAVLT)
   Prose Recall—The Lion Story
   Peabody Picture Vocabulary Test–Revised (PPVT-R)

These tests were given to subjects in Study 1 and are described in detail
in Felton et al. (1987). Additional language tests included:

   Rapid Alternating Stimulus (Wolf, 1984). Subjects are required
to name, as rapidly as possible, items presented visually on a chart.
The two-set Rapid Alternating Stimulus (RAS-A) task consists of five
letters and five numbers, repeated in a fixed A-B-A-B pattern. The three-
set task (RAS-B) consists of five letters, five numbers, and five colors,
repeated in a fixed A-B-C-A-B-C pattern.

   Phonological Awareness Tasks (Stanovich, Cunningham, &
Cramer, 1984). The "Final consonant different" task requires the subject

to listen to four words and choose the one that has a different ending sound. The "Strip initial consonant" task requires the subject to delete the initial phoneme of a word and pronounce the word that remains.

Syllable Counting Test (Mann & Liberman, 1984). The subject is required to listen to a series of one-, two-, and three-syllable words and tap out the number of syllables. Scores reflect errors.

The Lindamood Auditory Conceptualization Test (Lindamood & Lindamood, 1971). The subject manipulates wooden blocks of different colors to indicate speech sound patterns in two categories: isolated sounds in sequence and sounds within a syllable.

Word String Memory Test (Mann & Liberman, 1984). The subject is required to listen to strings of four words and to repeat the entire string in the exact order heard. Two sets of strings were given in a testing session (ST Memory 1 and ST Memory 2). In a modification of the original paradigm, only nonrhyming strings were scored for number correct rather than errors.

Tests of nonverbal functions:

Complex Figure Task (CFT) (Rey, 1964). The CFT is a measure of perceptual organization and visual memory in which the subject is instructed first to copy a complex figure, then to reproduce the figure from memory (immediate and delayed recall).

Judgment of Line Orientation (JL) (Benton, Hamsher, Varney, & Spreen, 1983). In this test, the subject is presented with 30 pairs of partial lines with each line corresponding to the orientation of one of the lines in a multiple choice response below it. The task is to determine which of the multiple choice lines corresponds exactly to each pair of partial lines.

Meier Visual Discrimination Test (Meier, personal communication, 1980). This test measures the ability to detect subtle similarities and differences among four sets of concentric circles, where the circles have randomly distributed gaps. The task is of theoretical interest because it contains no straight lines or angles, and can be considered a contrast to the JL test.

Raven Coloured Progressive Matrices (Raven, 1965). This test consists of a series of visual pattern matching and analogy problems pictured in nonrepresentational designs.

Test of sensorimotor function:

Finger Adduction Test (Kinsbourne & Caplan, 1979). This test requires subjects selectively to adduct any two adjacent fingers, without adducting the others. It is operationalized by placing a pencil between each pair of adjacent fingers, then pointing to the one to be selectively dropped, and measuring how many other fingers in either hand are also dropped.

3. Assessments of attention deficit disorder:

The Diagnostic Interview for Children and Adolescents–Parent Interview (Herjanic, 1983). See Study 1.

Classroom Behavior Inventory (Schaefer, Edgerton, & Aronson, 1977). The Classroom Behavior Inventory (CBI) is a 20-item questionnaire, filled out by the classroom teacher, that measures four bipolar attributes: independence versus dependence, task orientation versus distractibility, extroversion versus introversion, and considerateness versus hostility.

Conners Abbreviated Teacher Rating Scales (Goyette, Conners, & Ulrich, 1978). The abbreviated form is a revised version of the original Conners, consisting of 10 items on which the teacher rates each subject.

Procedures and Design.   Between November of the first grade and August prior to the second grade, each subject was tested individually with the above test battery. Testing required approximately 3 hours and was done in the school by a psychologist. In addition to testing of subjects, an attempt was made to conduct an interview with each child's parent or guardian. The interview concerned developmental, school, and family histories as well as the attention deficit disorder portion of the DICA. Interview information was obtained for 465 subjects. In the spring of the first grade, classroom teachers were asked to complete first the CBI and, 3 weeks later, the Conners on each child.

Given the age of the subjects in this study, we considered it inappropriate to attempt a definitive diagnosis of either ADD or RD. Rather, we chose to characterize subjects as to their relative degree of impairment on measures of attention and beginning reading skills in comparison to their peers. For attentional problems, this was operationalized in the following manner. The empirical distribution of total item scores on the DICA was cut at the 5th, 16th, and 84th percentiles—thus establishing four groups: respectively, "serious" (below fifth percentile in attentional control), "borderline" (from 5th to 16th percentiles), "normal" (from 16th to 84th percentiles), and "super-normal" (above 84th percentile). The concurrent validity of the DICA was established by correlation with teacher reports as assessed by the distractibility and task orientation factors of the CBI ($r = -.50$ and $.49$) and by the Abbreviated Conners Teachers Checklist ($r = -.47$).

Reading ability was assessed by the word identification subtest of the Woodcock-Johnson. Scores on this subtest were entered as dependent measures in a multiple regression with age, sex, and PPVT-R scores as predictors. The residuals from this regression then became the measures of specific reading ability as discrepant from PPVT-R IQ and as controlled for age and sex. Subjects were then classified on this discrepancy measure by the same procedure described above for the DICA: cutting at the 5th, 16th, and 84th percentiles to establish four groups of specific reading ability. The concurrent validity of this reading measure was assessed by correlation with the word identification score on the DST, which had also been corrected for age, sex, and PPVT-R. This correlation was .92.

Using these classifications, we selected two reading groups for comparison: the unambiguously impaired (below the 5th percentile) and the normal (between 16th and 84th percentiles). This resulted in an RD group of 25 subjects ($\overline{X}$ age = 7.14) and a NoRD group of 333 subjects ($\overline{X}$ age = 7.13) (see Table 5.5). Eliminating the borderline group insures a clean separation in reading ability; eliminating the super-normal group insures that any differences between impaired and normal are not due simply to the super-normal subjects. Attention deficit, however, was allowed to vary across all four levels or categories. Covariates (separate sources of predictable variance) were age, sex, PPVT-R as a measure of general verbal knowledge, and Raven Matrices as a measure of nonverbal problem-solving ability.

Results

Not surprisingly, the overall multivariate analysis of covariance shows that the combination of RD, ADD, age, sex, PPVT-R, and Raven Matrices was highly predictive of the set of cognitive dependent

TABLE 5.5
Subject Characteristics of RD and NoRD Samples

Variable	NoRD		RD	
	M	SD	M	SD
PPVT-R standard score	97.9	(18.1)	109.8	(14.4)
RPM raw score	20.2	(5.3)	18.6	(4.0)
Woodcock-Johnson word identification				
raw score	21.4	(4.5)	13.8	(2.2)
DICA total score	26.3	(4.6)	28.4	(4.8)
Conners score	6.2	(6.4)	11.9	(7.8)

Note. RD = reading disability; PPVT-R = Peabody Picture Vocabulary Test–Revised; DICA = Diagnostic Interview for Children and Adolescents; RPM = Raven Progressive Matrices.

measures ($p < .0001$). Of more specific interest is the separate impact on each cognitive dependent measure: Table 5.6 summarizes the univariate general linear model for each dependent measure. In this table, each predictor shows a p value for the prediction of each cognitive measure: These predictors are based upon Type III sums of squares, that is, on the unique variance attributable to that predictor, when all other predictors are held constant.

As in Study 1, these data show clear separation of ADD and RD effects. Once again, confrontation naming and rapid automatized naming are found to be strongly related to RD even when general ability factors are statistically controlled. In addition, two phonological awareness tasks (final consonant and strip consonant) are also significantly related to RD. Although the group differences on syllable counting and the Lindamood Test did not reach statistical significance ($p < .093$ and .054, respectively), the group with RD performed more poorly on both measures. On the word string memory test, the RD group performed less well than the NoRD group only on the second set of word strings. This set was administered later in the testing session, and the results may reflect a fatigue effect that was relatively greater for the subjects with RD. Figures 5.1 and 5.2 present the group profiles on these tasks. Number of false alarms on the recognition trial of the RAVLT was also significantly related to RD. Inspection of the data indicates that this effect was due to an unusually high number of false alarms by only 3 of the RD subjects.

To evaluate the amount of variance in reading ability explained by the several predictor and control variables, we calculated partial correlations between reading group (RD and NoRD) and each dependent measure, holding constant all other covariates. For the rapid naming variables, the partial correlations ranged from $-.30$ to $-.42$, with letter naming and the rapid alternating stimulus (RAS-B) accounting for the largest amount of variance (.42 in both cases). In contrast, the partial correlation between the Boston Naming Test and reading level was only .19. Partial correlations for the phonological awareness tests (final consonant and strip consonant) were .18 and .33, respectively. The word string memory test had a partial correlation of only .11.

The ADD effects, as in Study 1, are in the memory domain (delayed recall of the prose story and Trial 5 of the RAVLT) with additional effects on the Boston Naming Test, the strip initial consonant task, and the Meier visual similarity detection paradigm.

Discussion

This study is of special interest since it does not depend on a clinic-referred sample, or any other preselected criterion for accessing cases.

TABLE 5.6
Means, Standard Deviations, and Significant (<.05) p Values for Dependent Variables in General Linear Model

Dependent Variable	RD $\bar{x}$ (SD)	NoRD $\bar{x}$ (SD)	RD effect[a] p<	ADD effect[b] p<	PPVT-R p<	RPM p<
Finger Adduction	4.55 (3.71)	3.71 (3.03)	—	—	—	.0002
Prose Recall, Delayed	10.04 (4.88)	9.95 (4.23)	—	.0155	.0056	.0001
Figure Recall, Delayed	12.90 (5.84)	13.65 (5.96)	—	—	.0040	.0001
RAVLT Trial 1	5.28 (1.59)	4.97 (1.60)	—	—	.0001	—
RAVLT Trial 5	8.96 (2.70)	9.55 (2.51)	—	.0471	.0336	.0062
RAVLT Distractor Trial	4.40 (1.35)	4.23 (1.52)	—	—	.0001	—
RAVLT Postdistractor Trial	7.32 (3.29)	8.08 (2.48)	—	—	—	.061
RAVLT Misses	1.00 (1.44)	.93 (1.32)	—	—	—	—
RAVLT False Alarms	1.40 (2.99)	.48 (.94)	.0001	—	.0125	—
BNT	27.79 (6.37)	28.71 (7.19)	.0004	.0400	.0000	.0005
RAN–Colors	73.64 (26.36)	55.99 (15.94)	.0001	—	.0002	—
RAN–Number	61.28 (35.13)	40.49 (16.61)	.0001	—	.0001	—
RAN–Object	107.00 (31.18)	78.31 (24.93)	.0001	—	.0001	—
RAN–Letter	65.36 (39.08)	39.75 (12.35)	.0001	—	.0001	—
RAS–A	76.24 (28.23)	49.68 (16.83)	.0001	—	.0001	.0402
RAS–B	95.24 (37.37)	57.77 (21.00)	.0001	—	.0001	.0001
Lindamood	42.56 (16.30)	49.61 (22.17)	—	.0083	.0001	.0021
Strip Consonant	4.54 (4.22)	7.96 (2.96)	.0001	—	.0001	.0015
Final Consonant	5.00 (2.45)	6.45 (2.47)	.0010	—	.0003	.0040
Syllable Counting	7.72 (5.76)	6.28 (5.56)	—	—	.0006	—
Short-term Memory 1	12.48 (3.79)	12.23 (3.39)	—	—	.0004	—
Short-term Memory 2	10.28 (4.13)	11.41 (3.75)	.0495	.0038	.0007	—
Meier	8.60 (1.89)	9.25 (2.64)	—	—	.0001	.0001
Judgment of Line	6.32 (5.60)	6.82 (6.31)	—	—	.0329	.0001

Note: RD = reading disability; ADD = attention deficit disorder; RAVLT = Rey Auditory Verbal Learning Test; BNT = Boston Naming Test; RAN = Rapid Automatized Naming Tests; RAS = Rapid Alternating Stimulus.

[a] The RD effects are calculated for each dependent variable with Peabody Picture Vocabulary Test–Revised (PPVT-R), Raven Progressive Matrices (RPM), Sex, Age, and ADD category (levels 1 through 4) held constant as covariates.

[b] The ADD effects are calculated for each dependent variable with PPVT-R, RPM, Age, Sex, and RD category (RD and NoRD) held constant as covariates.

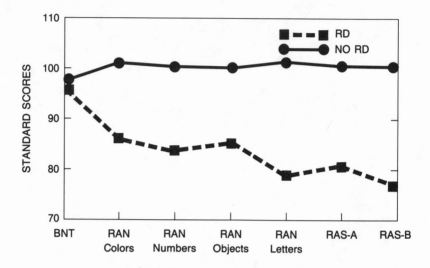

Figure 5.1. Performance of subjects with (RD) and without (NoRD) reading disabilities on confrontation and Rapid Automatized Naming Tests.

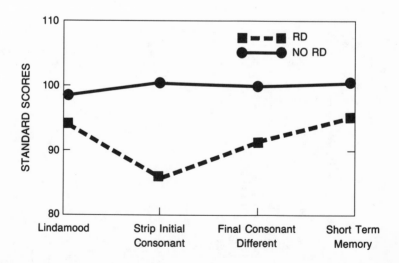

Figure 5.2. Performance of subjects with (RD) and without (NoRD) reading disabilities on phonological and verbal short-term memory tests.

Except for whatever self-selection bias there might have been for participation (and we are unaware of any systematic bias in this regard, since many of the cases were obtained only after long and persistent recruiting efforts), this sample can be considered representative of the breadth of the general population of public school first graders.

As such, the sample greatly strengthens the trend of the previous two studies in showing that separate accounting for ADD and RD improves the precision with which specific cognitive deficits can be attributed to each group. In particular, it replicates our own and others' findings of naming and phonemic awareness deficits in reading disability—findings that can now be considered secure from confounds by any level of ADD or by general verbal or nonverbal ability.

Perhaps the major new contribution of the study lies in the demonstration of these separable effects of RD and ADD in a sample as young as the first grade. Reading deficit (here operationalized as the degree to which word calling is discrepant from picture vocabulary as measured by the PPVT-R, age, and sex) is highly specific to naming and phonemic awareness deficits, and separable on most tasks from ADD, despite the youth and scholastic inexperience of the subjects: The effects are as strong for this age as for older subjects. Not only does this establish that the deficit is present and measurable at the initial stages of the school career, but it also shows that the general domain of accompanying deficit in naming and phonemic awareness is equally relevant for this age as it is for older students and even adults (Felton & Wood, 1988).

The ADD effects, as already illustrated in Study 2, are more variable and complex. The Meier visual task, with its demand for careful searching and its vulnerability to incomplete or impulsive analysis, is plausible as a marker for ADD, but it remains to be seen whether this task will continue to be vulnerable at later ages (no comparative data on this task are yet available). Moreover, while the memory domain is still implicated, it is particularly noteworthy and interesting that narrative prose recall is vulnerable in first graders, whereas it had been immune from ADD effects in older children (Study 1). We interpret this as suggesting that at this young age children cannot use the inherent structure of the story as a redundant protection against inattention, whereas in later years they can. This interpretation suggests that the vulnerability of specific tasks to attention deficit—unlike the vulnerability of specific tasks to the deficit constellation in reading disability—may vary across the years, as children learn various strategies for coping with their attentional problems. The moderate ADD effect on the Boston Naming Test was not found in the previous study of older children (Study 1) and, along with the effect on strip initial consonant, requires further study.

GENERAL CONCLUSIONS AND RECOMMENDATIONS

In this series of studies we have attempted to specify and separate the cognitive deficits associated with reading difficulties from those associated with attentional deficits. Our focus has been on a set of cognitive tasks of theoretical interest to the field of reading disabilities. In respect to these tasks, the effects of ADD and RD were quite different. The cognitive deficits associated with difficulties in reading were consistent across samples (school referred and randomly selected), developmental levels (beginning readers and upper-elementary-level students), and definitions and subtypes of reading disabilities. With IQ, age, and sex controlled for, subjects with RD were significantly impaired on measures of confrontation naming, rapid automatized naming, and phonological awareness. No consistent RD effects were found on measures of verbal learning and memory for lists of words presented over trials, memory for narrative material, or on tasks involving visual memory or visual perception. Consistent with numerous reports in the literature (Torgesen, in press), there was a moderate RD effect on the second administration of a word string memory task that requires verbatim recall of words in sequence.

Many questions remain, of course. Perhaps most important is the impact of environmental factors, especially teaching methods and treatment of ADD, on the acquisition of reading skills. As Calfee (1983) has suggested, current research fails to rule out the possibility that, for a considerable portion of children, reading disabilities "represent an instructional dysfunction rather than a constitutional disability" (p. 77). In addition, a recent study (Richardson, Kupietz, & Matinsky, 1987) indicates that effectiveness of pharmacological treatment is a critical factor in determining the response of ADD subjects to reading instruction.

In order to answer these questions, future studies will have to be much more comprehensive and inclusive than in the past. Subjects should represent the full range of reading and intellectual skills as well as socioeconomic levels in nonreferred samples and should be studied longitudinally from the earliest stages of reading acquisition. Given the well-documented problems with discrepancy models (McKinney, 1987; Rudel, 1985; Share, McGee, McKenzie, Williams, & Silva, 1987), such criteria should not be the sole basis for subject classification. The use of reading age controls will also be important for accurate interpretation of results.

The choice of research measures as well as design should be driven by theoretical considerations and based on models of reading disabilities. Tests of reading and spelling should be comprehensive and include measures of single word recognition, decoding and encoding of real and pseudowords, prose passage reading, and comprehension. Data should be gathered not only on errors but also on rate and automaticity. In addition to group comparisons, studies should include fine-grained analyses of individual subjects (e.g., Snowling, Stackhouse, & Rack, 1986). With large, nonreferred samples, it should be possible to identify subjects who are impaired on specific clusters of variables (e.g., naming, short-term memory, phonological awareness). These subjects should be followed longitudinally to determine the range of educational outcomes as well as the variability in the developmental course of these skills. It will be particularly informative to identify and study the full range of cognitive abilities in children who have deficits in one of these areas but who are not reading disabled.

Accurate assessment of attentional problems in reading disabled children as well as in control groups depends upon valid, reliable, and agreed-upon methods of defining and diagnosing the disorder. Given the inherent bias in referred samples of ADD children (e.g., Sandoval & Lambert, 1984–85), studies of ADD must also focus on nonreferred samples and should include children from the various subtypes that have been identified. Information should be gathered from different sources (i.e., parents, teachers, and self-report) as well as over time and across situations. Instruments must be validated on large samples of subjects across the age span from childhood to adulthood.

In addition to suggesting directions for future research, the studies reported here have educational implications. First, it is clear that significant differences in basic processing abilities important for the development of adequate reading skills are present and quantifiable from the very beginning of children's academic experience. This leads to the obvious need for early identification and appropriate instruction prior to the development of reading problems severe enough to meet standard learning disability criteria. Second, the consistent finding of the relationship of both phonological processing and rapid naming abilities to the development of good reading skills suggests that these areas should be addressed educationally. Research by Bradley and Bryant (1985) demonstrating that direct instruction in phonological awareness improves reading skills, as well as numerous studies (see Perfetti, 1985, for a review) indicating the importance of an adequate knowledge of decoding principles for the development of fluent reading and comprehension, suggests that beginning reading instruction should make these principles explicit. Automaticity in word recognition is also vital and may, particularly in children with retrieval problems, require extremely high levels of overlearning and practice. An instructional program that incorporates direct teaching of the alphabetic code, coupled with techniques designed to develop automaticity, appears to be a reasonable first step. To be maximally effec-

110   FELTON AND WOOD

tive, such instruction should be an integral part of the basal reading curriculum from the beginning of reading instruction rather than a peripheral remedial effort offered after failure.

REFERENCES

Ackerman, P.T., Anhalt, J.M., Dykman, R.A., & Holcomb, P.J. (1986). Effortful processing deficits in children with reading and/or attention disorders. *Brain and Cognition, 5,* 22–40.

Ackerman, P.T., & Dykman, R.A. (1982). Automatic and effortful information-processing deficits in children with learning and attention disorders. *Topics in Learning & Learning Disabilities, 2,* 12–22.

Ackerman, P.T., Dykman, R.A., & Oglesby, D.M. (1983). Sex and group differences in reading and attention disordered children with and without hyperkinesis. *Journal of Learning Disabilities, 16,* 407–415.

Barnes, T., & Forness, S. (1982). Learning characteristics of children and adolescents with various psychiatric diagnoses. In R. Rutherford (Ed.), *Severe behavior disorders of children and youth* (pp. 32–41). Reston, VA: Council for Children with Behavior Disorders.

Benton, A.L., & Hamsher, K. de S. (1976). *Multilingual aphasia examination.* Iowa City: University of Iowa.

Benton, A.L., Hamsher, K. de S., Varney, N.R., & Spreen, O. (1983). *Contributions to neuropsychological assessment.* New York: Oxford University Press.

Blachman, B.A. (1983). Are we assessing the linguistic factors critical in early reading? *Annals of Dyslexia, 33,* 91–110.

Boder, E., & Jarrico, S. (1982). *The Boder test of reading/spelling patterns.* New York: Grune & Stratton.

Bohline, D.S. (1985). Intellectual and affective characteristics of attention deficit disordered children. *Journal of Learning Disabilities, 18,* 604–608.

Bradley, L., & Bryant, P. (1985). *Rhyme and reason in reading and spelling.* Ann Arbor: University of Michigan Press.

Calfee, R. (1983). Book review of Dyslexia: Theory and research by F.R. Vellutino. *Applied Psycholinguistics, 4,* 69–101.

Cantwell, D.P., & Satterfield, J.H. (1978). The prevalence of academic underachievement in hyperactive children. *Journal of Pediatric Psychology, 24,* 161–171.

Chapman, L.J., & Chapman, J.P. (1973). Problems in the measurement of cognitive deficit. *Psychological Bulletin, 79,* 380–385.

Denckla, M.B., & Rudel, R.G. (1976). Naming of object drawings by dyslexic and other learning disabled children. *Brain and Language, 3,* 1–16.

Douglas, V.I., & Peters, K.G. (1979). Toward a clearer definition of the attentional deficit of hyperactive children. In G.A. Hale & M. Lewis (Eds.), *Attention and cognitive development.* New York: Plenum Press.

Dunn, L.M., & Dunn, L.M. (1981). *Peabody picture vocabulary test–Revised.* Circle Pines, MN: American Guidance Service.

Dykman, R.A., Ackerman, P.T., & Holcomb, P.J. (1985). Reading disabled and ADD children: Similarities and differences. In D. Gray & J. Kavanaugh (Eds.), *Biobehavioral measures of dyslexia* (pp. 47–69). Parkton, MD: York Press.

Dykman, R.A., Ackerman, P.T., Holcomb, P.J., & Bondreau, Y. (1983). Physiological manifestations of learning disability. In G.M. Senf & J.K. Torgesen (Eds.), *Annual review of learning disabilities* (pp. 80–87). Chicago: Journal of Learning Disabilities.

Felton, R.H., & Wood, F.B. (1988). *Cognitive phenotype of adult dyslexia.* Manuscript submitted for publication.

Felton, R.H., Wood, F.B., Brown, I.B., Campbell, S.K., & Harter, M.R. (1987). Separate verbal memory and naming deficits in attention deficit disorder and reading disability. *Brain and Language, 31,* 171–184.

Fleisher, L.S., Soodak, L.C., & Jelin, M.A. (1984). Selective attention deficits in learning disabled children: Analysis of the data base. *Exceptional Children, 51,* 136–141.

Goyette, C.H., Conners, C.K., & Ulrich, R.F. (1978). Normative data on revised Conners parent and teacher rating scales. *Journal of Abnormal Child Psychology, 6,* 221–236.

Halperin, J.M., Gittelman, R., Klein, D.F., & Rudel, G. (1984). Reading-disabled hyperactive children: A distinct subgroup of attention deficit disorder with hyperactivity? *Journal of Abnormal Child Psychology, 12,* 1–14.

Herjanic, B. (1983). *The Washington University diagnostic interview for children and adolescents.* St. Louis, MO: Washington University Medical Center.

Holobrow, P.L., & Berry, P.S. (1986). Hyperactivity and learning difficulties. *Journal of Learning Disabilities, 19,* 426–431.

Hooper, S.C., & Hynd, G.W. (1985). Differential diagnosis of developmental dyslexia with the Kaufman Assessment Battery for Children (K-ABC). *Journal of Clinical Child Psychology, 14,* 145–152.

Kaplan, E., Goodglass, H., & Weintraub, S. (1982). *Boston naming test.* Philadelphia: Lea & Fiebiger.

Kinsbourne, M. (1982). The role of selective attention in reading disability. In R.N. Malatesha & P.G. Aaron (Eds.), *Reading disorder—Varieties and treatments* (pp. 199–214). New York: Academic Press.

Kinsbourne, M., & Caplan, P.J. (1979). *Children's learning and attention problems.* Boston: Little, Brown.

Koppell, S. (1979). Testing the attentional deficit notion. *Journal of Learning Disabilities, 12,* 52–57.

Krupski, A. (1986). Attention problems in youngsters with learning handicaps. In J.K. Torgesen & B.Y.L. Wong (Eds.), *Psychological and educational perspectives on learning disabilities* (pp. 161–192). New York: Academic Press.

Lahey, B.B., Stempniak, M., Robinson, E.J., & Tyroler, M. (1978). Hyperactivity and learning disabilities as independent dimensions of child behavior problems. *Journal of Abnormal Psychology, 87,* 333–340.

Lambert, N.M., & Sandoval, J. (1980). The prevalence of learning disabilities in a sample of children considered hyperactive. *Journal of Abnormal Child Psychology, 8,* 33–50.

Levine, M.D., Busch, B., & Aufsuser, C. (1982). The dimension of inattention among children with school problems. *Pediatrics, 70,* 387–395.

Lezak, M.D. (1983). *Neuropsychological assessment.* New York/Oxford: Oxford University Press.

Liberman, I.Y. (1983). A language-oriented view of reading and its disabilities. In H.R. Myklebust (Ed.), *Progress in learning disabilities* (pp. 81–102). New York: Grune & Stratton.

Lindamood, C.H., & Lindamood, P.C. (1971). *Lindamood auditory conceptualization test.* Boston: Teaching Resources Corp.

Mann, V.A., & Liberman, I.Y. (1984). Phonological awareness and verbal short-term memory: Can they presage early reading problems? *Journal of Learning Disabilities, 17,* 592–599.

McKinney, J.D. (1987). Research on the identification of learning-disabled children: Perspectives on changes in educational policy. In S. Vaughn & C.S. Bos (Eds.), *Research in learning disabilities: Issues and future directions* (pp. 215–238). Boston: Little, Brown.

Olson, R.K. (1985). Disabled reading process and cognitive profiles. In D. Gray & J. Kavanaugh (Eds.), *Biobehavioral measures of dyslexia* (pp. 215–243). Parkton, MD: York Press.

Perfetti, C.A. (1985). *Reading ability.* New York: Oxford University Press.

Raven, J.C. (1965). *Guide to using the Coloured Progressive Matrices.* London: H.K. Lewis.

Rey, A. (1964). *L'examen clinique en psychologie.* Paris: Presses Universitaires de France.

Richardson, E., & DeBenedetto, B. (1985). *The decoding skills test.* Parkton, MD: York Press.

Richardson, E., Kupietz, S., & Matinsky, S. (1987). Considerations in the treatment of development reading disorder in hyperactive children. In J. Loney (Ed.), *The young hyperactive child.* Boston: Hayworth.

Rudel, R.G. (1985). The definition of dyslexia: Language and motor deficits. In F.H. Duffy & N. Geschwind (Eds.), *Dyslexia: A neuroscientific approach to clinical evaluation.* Boston: Little, Brown.

Sandoval, J., & Lambert, N.M. (1984–85). Hyperactive and learning disabled children: Who gets help? *The Journal of Special Education, 18,* 495–503.

Schaefer, E.S., Edgerton, M., & Aronson, M. (1977). *Classroom behavior inventory.* Chapel Hill, NC: Frank Porter Graham Child Development Center.

Share, D.L., McGee, R., McKenzie, D., Williams, S., & Silva, P.A. (1987). Further evidence relating to the distinction between specific reading retardation and general reading backwardness. *British Journal of Developmental Psychology, 5,* 35–44.

Shaywitz, S.E. (1986). *Early recognition of educational vulnerability: A technical report.* Hartford, CT: State Department of Education.

Snowling, M., Stackhouse, I., & Rack, J. (1986). Phonological dyslexia and dysgraphia —A developmental analysis. *Cognitive Neuropsychology, 3,* 309–339.

Stanovich, K.E., Cunningham, A.E., & Cramer, B.B. (1984). Assessing phonological awareness in kindergarten children: Issues of task comparability. *Journal of Experimental Child Psychology, 38,* 175–190.

Talland, G.A. (1965). *Deranged memory.* New York: Academic Press.

Taylor, E.M. (1959). *The appraisal of children with cerebral deficits.* Cambridge, MA: Harvard University Press.

Torgesen, J.K. (in press). Studies of learning disabled children who perform poorly on memory span tasks. *Journal of Learning Disabilities.*

Van den Bos, K.P. (1984). Letter processing in dyslexic subgroups. *Annals of Dyslexia,* *34,* 179–194.

Vellutino, F.R. (1983). Childhood dyslexia: A language disorder. In H.R. Myklebust (Ed.), *Progress in learning disabilities* (pp. 135–173). New York: Grune & Stratton.

Vellutino, F.R., & Scanlon, D.M. (1982). Verbal processing in poor and normal readers. In P.S. Branerd & N. Pressley (Eds.), *Verbal processes in children.* New York: Springer-Verlag.

Wolf, M. (1984). Naming, reading, and the dyslexias: A longitudinal overview. *Annals of Dyslexia, 34,* 87–115.

Woodcock, R.W., & Johnson, M.B. (1977). *Woodcock-Johnson psycho-educational battery.* Hingham, MA: Teaching Resources.

6. Longitudinal Research on the Behavioral Characteristics of Children with Learning Disabilities

JAMES D. McKINNEY

Prospective longitudinal research on children with learning disabilities is rare (Kavale, 1988; McKinney & Feagans, 1984). Although an exten-sive literature has evolved that describes the cognitive, linguistic, and behavioral differences between children with learning disabilities (LD) and normally achieving peers, we still have little understanding about how these differences emerge developmentally, change over time, and contribute to academic failure. Most of the evidence on the prognosis for children with learning disabilities comes from follow-up studies of clinical samples (Gottesman, 1979; Horn, O'Donnell, & Vitulano, 1983) or from prospective studies of high-risk samples (Werner & Smith, 1977). Although most follow-up studies are seriously flawed by a variety of sampling and methodological problems, the bulk of the evidence points to an unfavorable prognosis—continued academic failure and elevated risk for behavioral and adjustment problems (Deshler, 1978; Gresham, 1988; Thompson, 1986; Werner & Smith, 1977).

This research was supported by grants from the National Institute of Child Health and Human Development (HD07178) and the Department of Education, OSEP (Nos. G00843005 and G00780285). The author gratefully acknowledges the contributions of his colleagues Lynne Feagans, Deborah Speece, and Mark Appelbaum in the development and execution of this research program.

At the same time, there are marked individual differences in achievement outcomes for children with LD that remain largely unexplained (Kavale, 1988). Although several characteristics, such as ability level, socioeconomic status, and self-esteem, have been associated with academic outcomes for children with LD (Kavale, 1988), it is important both theoretically and practically to demonstrate such relationships prospectively rather than retrospectively. Evidence from longitudinal studies of children who are at risk for a variety of developmental disorders suggests that some high-risk children develop personal and social competencies that make them more resilient to stress and responsive to intervention (Farran & McKinney, 1986). If such characteristics could be identified early in the school experience of children with learning disabilities, and were shown to predict later outcomes, the potential would exist for improving diagnostic and special education practices, and perhaps for the prevention of social and emotional sequelae associated with persistent school failure.

The purpose of this chapter is to summarize the collective findings from the Carolina Learning Disabilities Research Program with respect to behavioral characteristics. The broad aims of this research program over the past 10 years have been (a) to provide a more comprehensive portrait of the development of children with learning disabilities during the elementary school years and (b) to determine the relationship between specific developmental processes and academic progress.

In order to pursue these aims, we began a program of cross-sectional research at the Frank Porter Graham Child Development Center in the mid-1970s that led to a larger longitudinal effort beginning in 1978. In the longitudinal study, we followed a sample of children identified as LD in the first and second grades for 3 years and compared their development to that of a randomly selected sample of average achievers. Subsequently, we conducted a follow-up study on the academic outcomes for children in the original longitudinal sample who were available when they reached the fifth and sixth grades. Although this research also provided evidence on cognitive and linguistic processes (Feagans, 1983; Feagans & Appelbaum, 1986; Feagans & Short, 1984; McKinney, Short, & Feagans, 1985), the present chapter focuses on findings with respect to behavioral characteristics.

Since theory in the field of learning disabilities has been influenced greatly by the concept of specific ability deficits and the neurological bases of the condition (Ramey & McKinney, 1981; Torgesen, 1975; Wong, 1979), most of the research on learning disabilities has focused on cognitive and linguistic processes. However, in the late 1970s, evidence began to converge on the classroom behavior of children with LD as a significant factor in explaining underachievement (McKinney & Feagans, 1983).

In summarizing our research on behavioral characteristics, I first briefly review the early studies that provided the theoretical rationale and methods used in subsequent longitudinal research, as well as our earlier cross-sectional studies. The longitudinal findings and subsequent work on the classification and validation of behavioral subtypes are described in greater depth, and are followed by a discussion of the implications of this research for theory and practice.

BACKGROUND AND PRELIMINARY STUDIES

Our longitudinal research on the behavioral characteristics of children with learning disabilities evolved from earlier correlational studies on the relationship between classroom behavior and academic achievement. These initial studies suggested that many of the behaviors attributed to children with LD (Bryan, 1974; Bryan & Wheeler, 1972; Forman & McKinney, 1975; Forness & Esveldt, 1975) were also associated with academic achievement generally (Hoge & Luce, 1979). Collectively, studies of general education samples suggested that students who were attentive, independent, and who interacted in a task-oriented fashion during instruction were more likely to succeed academically than those who were distractible, dependent, and poorly task oriented (Hoge & Luce, 1979).

Early Observational Studies

McKinney, Mason, Perkerson, and Clifford (1975) observed 90 second-grade students in general education settings during the fall and spring of the school year and took group-administered measures of achievement and general ability. Classroom behavior was measured by the Schedule for Classroom Activity Norms (SCAN), which was later adopted for research on children with LD. SCAN is a 12-category, point-time sampling method for coding task-oriented behavior, peer interaction, teacher interaction, and various types of problem behavior (aggression, dependency, gross motor inappropriate behavior, and nonconstructive self-directed activity).

McKinney et al. (1975) found multiple Rs of .63 and .51 between 12 SCAN variables and concurrent achievement scores. Predicting from fall to spring, IQ accounted for 49% of the variance in achievement scores, whereas behavior accounted for 36%. When behavior was added to IQ, the R^2 was increased to .76. Thus, classroom behavior provided significant information that was relatively independent of that provided by general ability. Significant behaviors in predicting spring achievement were passive responding, dependency, and distractibility, although constructive self-directed activity and aggression also predicted concurrently.

Subsequent studies with SCAN (Moore, Haskins, & McKinney, 1980; Oxford, Morrison, & McKinney, 1980; Richey & McKinney, 1978) demonstrated the effects of classroom contextual setting on behavior. For example, Richey and McKinney (1978) found that differences in distractibility between boys with LD and classroom peers varied with the size of instructional groups and the presence or absence of teachers during instructional activities.

Teacher Perceptions of Classroom Behavior

During the same period of time, Schaefer (1981) developed a hierarchical model for adaptive classroom behavior as indexed by teacher ratings on the Classroom Behavior Inventory (CBI) (Schaefer, Edgerton, & Aronson, 1977). Factor analytic studies showed that the CBI measured three basic dimensions of adaptive behavior: academic competence as defined by ratings of verbal intelligence, independence and dependence, task orientation, and distractibility; personal adjustment as defined by ratings of extroversion/introversion; and social competence as defined by ratings of considerateness and hostility. Schaefer (1981) has shown significant relationships between teacher ratings on the CBI and achievement, both concurrently and longitudinally, as well as relationships between parent ratings of child behavior and parent beliefs and attitudes about schooling.

More importantly, for the purposes of our research, Schaefer's (1981) model suggested specific hypotheses about the behaviors teachers attribute to children with learning disabilities that distinguish them from children with mental retardation and those with emotional/behavioral disorders.

Subsequent research with the CBI showed consistent differences between children with LD and classmates, particularly with respect to teachers' perceptions of task-oriented behavior, independence, and verbal intelligence (Feagans & McKinney, 1981; Forman & McKinney, 1975; McKinney, McClure, & Feagans, 1982). Also, McKinney and Forman (1982) found that children identified as learning disabled, educable mentally retarded, and emotionally/behaviorally handicapped were discriminated by the CBI before they were identified by psychoeducational evaluation.

As part of this early work with SCAN and the CBI, we were able to replicate Schaefer's factor structure and to show conceptually consistent correlations between CBI scales and SCAN categories (McKinney & Feagans, 1980). Also, significant correlations were obtained between ratings of special education teachers and classroom teachers for children with learning disabilities across several samples. Finally, contrary to expectation, we found little evidence for gender differences on behavioral measures within samples of children with LD (Feagans & McKinney, 1980; McKinney et al., 1982), although girls performed more poorly on IQ and math tests.

CROSS-SECTIONAL RESEARCH

Initial methodological studies with SCAN and the CBI provided preliminary evidence on the validity of our general hypothesis about the role of classroom behavior as an important correlate of achievement with two conceptually related but different measures. However, the problem remained to link classroom behavior to the performance of children with LD specifically.

Accordingly, we conducted a series of cross-sectional studies to better demonstrate and replicate group effects. In general, cross-sectional comparisons between students with LD and randomly selected classmates yielded a consistent and comparable pattern of results when both observations and teacher ratings were obtained (Feagans & McKinney, 1981; McKinney & Feagans, 1980, 1983; McKinney et al., 1982). Classroom teachers rated students with LD less favorably than average achievers on task orientation/distractibility, independence/dependence, verbal intelligence, and creativity/curiosity. Typically in these studies, differences were not found on teacher ratings of considerateness/hostility, and the effects for extroversion/introversion were equivocal across studies.

Similarly, SCAN observations showed that students with LD displayed more off-task behavior overall, less on-task behavior in independent work, and more teacher interaction. With respect to academic performance, Feagans and McKinney (1981) found significant grade level (1 through 3) by group interactions, suggesting that the performance of students with LD became progressively poorer relative to the performance of classmates as they advanced in grades, and that this effect was upheld when IQ and parent education were covaried.

Subsequently, McKinney and Feagans (1980) found the same pattern of differences on CBI teacher ratings and SCAN observations between children with LD who were assessed 1 year later and a new group of randomly selected classmates. Also, students with LD failed to show significant gains on achievement tests between the first- and second-year assessments. Using the same follow-up data, McKinney and Speece (1983) evaluated the relative contribution of IQ, age, and classroom behavior in predicting residual gains in reading achievement from the first year to the second. Although SCAN observational data did not predict achievement gains, teachers' ratings on the academic competence and socialization factors of the CBI were significant predictors of gains in reading achievement for students with LD. In this regard, IQ and age were better predictors of reading comprehension concurrently, whereas classroom behavior ratings were better predictors of decoding skill both concurrently and longitudinally.

Teacher-Student Interaction

Given the consistent finding with SCAN that children with LD interacted more frequently with classroom teachers than did their classmates in instructional settings, it became important to describe the nature of such interaction under the general hypothesis that distractibility and disruptive behavior elicit the attention of teachers. Dorval, McKinney, and Feagans (1982) recorded dialogues between 12 classroom teachers and first- and second-grade children with LD and randomly selected classmates without LD.

Teachers initiated interactions more frequently with students with LD, and the majority of the dialogues (63%) pertained to behavior management. These dialogues occurred primarily in response to student inattention and rule infraction, which were more likely to occur in whole class rather than small group activities. Also, learning disabled students' initiations to teachers were more often situationally inappropriate. On the other hand, the students with LD received comparable numbers of instructional and social initiations from teachers, suggesting that the students with LD were not ignored in this regard. These findings, together with those from SCAN observations, tend to support teachers' perceptions of student behavior, and in part explain their grouping practices for students with LD.

LONGITUDINAL RESEARCH

Research conducted to this point showed that as a heterogeneous group, children with LD displayed maladaptive patterns of classroom behavior that distinguished them from normally achieving classmates and were associated with their failure to progress academically. However, the implications of these studies were limited by the correlative nature of cross-sectional group comparisons and by the absence of evidence that maladaptive behavior contributed to academic retardation developmentally. Thus, in the absence of longitudinal evidence, we could not infer that the greater disparity between the achievement of children with LD and their normally achieving classmates at higher grade levels actually represented a progressive decline in relative performance. In the same vein, we could not conclude that consistent patterns of differences between children with LD and classmates at different age levels represented developmental continuity with respect to these characteristics.

Methodological Considerations

Several methodological factors should be noted with respect to our longitudinal results. These factors include the sample selection procedure, sample attrition, and the effects of changes in the definition of learning disabilities since the implementation of P.L. 94-142.

Research Sample.   The initial sample of students with LD was drawn from all newly identified first- and second-grade students in a large school system, and each child was enrolled in special education within 6 weeks of identification. We deliberately chose young, newly identified children because we wished to monitor progress from the onset of special education before children had a long history of school failure. Children with Wechsler Intelligence Scale for Children–Revised (WISC-R) (Wechsler, 1974) IQs below 85 were eliminated from the study. In addition to socioeconomic and psychometric data, we took detailed histories from parents and school records.

Comparison students were randomly selected from the pool of same-sex and same-race average achievers in each mainstream classroom that contained a participant with LD. Normal ability and achievement were verified for comparison children by individual tests. Although black children were somewhat overrepresented, there were no differences in socioeconomic level between the groups, and the full range of socioeconomic levels was represented. Parent permission to participate was obtained in over 95% of the cases. A more complete description of sample characteristics can be found in McKinney and Feagans (1984).

Sample Attrition.   Children were followed with cognitive, linguistic, and behavioral measures for 3 years, until they reached 8 to 9 years of age.

When they reached the age of 11-6 years we conducted a follow-up study that involved 42 pairs of the original 63 pairs of learning disabled and average achieving students. Eight learning disabled and six comparison students were lost to attrition over the first 3-year period of the project, and another 20 were lost by the end-point assessment at 11-6 years. Tests comparing the reduced sample to the original sample showed no evidence of selective attrition.

Effects of Changes in Identification Criteria.   The longitudinal sample was drawn in 1978/79 during the implementation of P.L. 94-142 and children were identified on the basis of age/grade discrepancy in achievement and a psychological evaluation to provide evidence of process disability. A major change over the course of the project was the use of IQ/achievement discrepancy criteria to determine eligibility for services.

Accordingly, we conducted additional studies to determine the effects of new discrepancy criteria on the characteristics and outcomes for the sample (McKinney, 1987; Short, Feagans, McKinney, & Appelbaum, 1986). Based on first-year IQ and achievement data, we found that 40% of the children with LD were significantly discrepant, whereas 23% of the comparison sample were discrepant. Status as discrepant was unrelated to subject variables and socioeconomic level. The magnitude of IQ/achievement discrepancy increased for the children with LD over the course of the study but was quite stable for comparison children (Short et al., 1986). Finally, initial status as discrepant was unrelated to student outcomes for either children with LD or comparison children (McKinney, 1987). Thus, we have no evidence that changes in the identification criteria with respect to IQ/achievement discrepancy had any significant effect on the longitudinal data of interest in this study, although it is always questionable whether the findings would represent those that might be obtained with contemporary samples.

Longitudinal Results

The results with respect to longitudinal trends for group comparisons on achievement and behavioral measures are described below. A more detailed description of these results can be found in McKinney and Feagans (1984).

Academic Achievement.   Figure 6.1 shows the longitudinal trend for students with LD and comparison students over the first 3 years of the project as measured by Peabody Individual Achievement Test

(PIAT) (Dunn & Markwardt, 1970) scores. Multivariate repeated measures analysis showed that compared to average achievers, children with LD (a) tended to maintain their same relative status on reading recognition, (b) showed a significant linear decline in reading comprehension, and (c) improved slightly in math and then declined.

A significant group × age interaction for the omnibus MANOVA supported the conclusion that the developmental trend overall for students with LD was one of progressive decline relative to comparison students. The full impact of this trend was evident in the follow-up assessment in the fifth and sixth grades with the Woodcock-Johnson Achievement Test (Woodcock & Johnson, 1977). At this point in time, the overall performance of students with LD was at the 23rd percentile for age, while that for comparison students was at the 49th percentile (McKinney & Feagans, 1988).

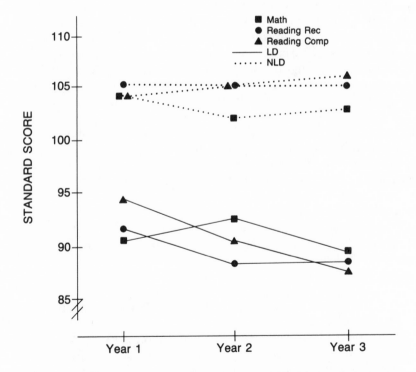

Figure 6.1. Longitudinal trends in mean Peabody Individual Achievement Test (PIAT) age standard scores. *Note.* From "Academic and Behavioral Characteristics: Longitudinal Studies of Learning Disabled Children and Average Achievers" by J.D. McKinney & L. Feagans, 1984, *Learning Disability Quarterly, 7,* p. 259. Copyright 1984 by the Council for Learning Disabilities. Reprinted by permission.

Classroom Behavior Inventory.   The patterns of CBI ratings given by three different sets of classroom teachers over the course of the project were remarkably similar. Although highly significant group effects were obtained each year that replicated cross-sectional studies (Feagans & McKinney, 1981), no significant change in teachers' perceptions from year to year was found. Classroom teachers consistently rated children with LD less favorably on all positive and negative scales of the CBI except considerateness and hostility. CBI ratings on children with LD were also obtained longitudinally from special education teachers. As in previous studies, we found significant correlations between the ratings of special education and classroom teachers as well as highly similar profile patterns.

SCAN Observational Data.   Initial group differences for on-task behavior, off-task behavior, and teacher interaction replicated earlier findings. Although there were no longitudinal changes in teacher ratings, there was substantial change in child behavior. However, for the most part, changes in the behavior of children with LD were offset by similar changes in the behavior of comparison children that tended to preserve the same relative differences in behavior that were observed initially. The analysis of the longitudinal trends indicated that although children with LD showed decreases in off-task behavior, the comparison children did, too. On the other hand, whereas comparison children showed a decrease in the frequency of teacher interaction and increases in on-task behavior in individual work, children with LD tended to maintain the same relative status on these behaviors.

Although no differences were found between groups, peer interaction, work preparation, dependency, and aggression decreased with advances in grade level. These data may explain the finding that different teachers in succeeding years failed to perceive changes in classroom behavior and suggest that in comparing students with LD and classmates, "the more things change, the more they stay the same."

LONGITUDINAL RESEARCH ON BEHAVIORAL SUBTYPES

Although the longitudinal assessment of group effects yielded new information about the academic and behavioral outcomes for children with LD, the most significant implications of the results were still obscured by the problem of sample heterogeneity (McKinney, 1984, 1988). For example, it would not be appropriate at this stage of the research to conclude that all children with LD show declining patterns of academic performance, or that the pattern of behavior illustrated by group means represents a distinct syndrome that characterizes learning disability, or for that matter, the behavior of any given individual in the sample.

Similarly, although teachers did not characterize children with LD as having conduct or severe personality problems, as a group, there is other evidence that emotional/behavior problems, attention problems, and learning disabilities coexist for significant numbers of children (Cullinan, Epstein, & Denbinski, 1979; Thompson, 1986). For example, there is ample reason to hypothesize a relationship between attentional disorders and conduct problems. Also, it is feasible that some children with LD would present a behavior pattern with high introversion and low task orientation that might have a motivational basis rather than an intrinsic neurological basis. Finally, it is also possible that some children with LD are developmentally normal with respect to behavioral characteristics and that they underachieve for other reasons (McKinney, 1984, 1988).

If such patterns of intraindividual differences could be related to students' academic progress longitudinally, it would be possible to posit a theory of risk for poor outcome that would guide the selection of more appropriate treatments for individual students. Also, if such patterns of behavior were prognostic of later outcome, we would have an empirical rationale for developing interventions to prevent later negative consequences.

In recent years, considerable progress has been made in the application of cluster analysis and other empirical classification techniques to subdivide heterogeneous samples of children with LD into more homogeneous subtypes based on their common characteristics (McKinney, 1988). Most of these studies have used neuropsychological and psychoeducational test batteries (Lyon, 1985; Rourke, 1985; Satz, Morris, & Fletcher, 1985), although some evidence is available on personality patterns (Porter & Rourke, 1985) and clinical subgroups (Achenbach & Edelbrock, 1981).

Classification of Behavioral Subtypes

To better describe the specific behavioral patterns displayed by children with LD, Speece, McKinney, and Appelbaum (1985) used hierarchical cluster analysis techniques to empirically classify subtypes within the original longitudinal sample of 63 children. Classroom teacher ratings were used to identify more homogeneous clusters of children with LD that differed primarily in profile shape, thereby reflecting the relative strengths and weaknesses of the children in each subtype. Also, Speece et al. used two different algorithms to select the "best" of alternative solutions and split sample replication and forecasting techniques to assess the internal validity of the solution. However, external validation is perhaps the most critical issue in cluster studies (Lyon, 1983; McKinney, 1988) because it is possible to get stable clusters of random data that have no theoretical or practical real world implications (Speece, 1988). In the present study, we used longitudinal measures of CBI ratings by special education teachers, SCAN observations, and achievement measures to externally validate the clusters formed on classroom teacher ratings.

Cluster Description

The mean cluster profiles standardized to the comparison sample are shown in Figure 6.2. The description and proportional membership of each are as follows:

Cluster 1. Attention Deficit (28.6%): This subtype showed deficiencies in task-oriented behavior and independence but displayed normal personal/social behavior.

Cluster 2. Normal Behavior (25.4%): Although this subtype showed slightly elevated ratings on considerateness and introversion, all profile points were within ±1 SD of the comparison means.

Cluster 3. Conduct Problems (14.3%): These children displayed mild attention deficits combined with elevated hostility and distractibility.

Cluster 4. Withdrawn Behavior (11%): This cluster was composed primarily of girls with LD and was rated as overly dependent and introverted.

Cluster 5. Normal Behavior (9.5%): Like Cluster 2, all the profile points for this subtype were in the normal range, but with slightly elevated ratings on hostility.

Cluster 6. Low Positive Behavior (6.3%): Children in this small subgroup showed uniformly low ratings on all positive behaviors but no corresponding elevation on negative behaviors.

Cluster 7. Global Behavior Problems (4.8%): This very small subgroup of 3 boys was rated as significantly impaired on all classroom behaviors.

External Validation

Two independent measures of classroom behavior were used to establish the external validity of the cluster descriptions. The first was

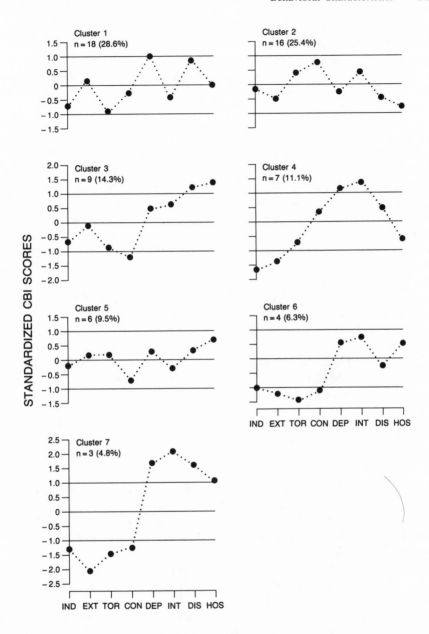

Figure 6.2. Mean cluster plots for behavioral subtypes. *Note.* From "Classification and Validation of Behavioral Subtypes of Learning Disabled Children" by D.L. Speece, J.D. McKinney, & M.I. Appelbaum, 1985, *Journal of Educational Psychology, 77,* p. 71. Copyright 1985 by the *Journal of Educational Psychology.* Reprinted by permission. (IND = independence; EXT = extroversion; TOR = task orientation; CON = considerateness; DEP = dependence; INT = introversion; DIS = distractibility; HOS = hostility.)

CBI ratings by special education teachers. Classroom teachers' and special education teachers' ratings for the first year of the study were standardized separately and are plotted in Figure 6.3 for the children in each cluster. As Figure 6.3 shows, profile shapes were consistent across clusters for the two groups of teachers with some minor variations in elevation.

In the second validation analysis, a priori hypotheses were generated to predict differences on specific categories of observed classroom behavior as measured by SCAN. The omnibus multivariate tests for conceptually similar behaviors (e.g., task-oriented and problem behavior) were all significant. Although contrasts among clusters were not significant for teacher and peer interaction, significant effects in the direction predicted were obtained between "normal appearing" clusters and atypical clusters, and among three of the five atypical clusters on measures of off-task behavior, gross motor inappropriate behavior, and aggression. A more complete description of these findings can be found in Speece et al. (1985).

Analysis of WISC-R IQ scores showed no differences among clusters. While the small number within clusters precluded valid chi-square tests, boys appeared to be overrepresented in the attention deficit and conduct problem clusters, and girls were somewhat overrepresented in the normal and withdrawn clusters. Also, parent education level appeared to be higher in the behaviorally normal LD subtypes than in atypical subtypes.

Longitudinal Stability

The longitudinal data on behavioral subtypes and their relationships to academic progress were based on complete data available at the end of 3 years on 47 children with LD (McKinney & Speece, 1986). Analyses by group and original subtype membership did not indicate selective attrition. Two different approaches were used to assess continuity in subtype membership over a 3-year period. The first pertains to the stability of the profile patterns themselves and the second to individual changes in classification.

To assess the stability of subtype membership, we used the forecasting technique to classify children who were rated on the CBI in Years 2 and 3 according to their original subtype membership in the first year. This technique uses the discriminant functions from the Year 1 clusters to predict subtype membership in subsequent years with new CBI data, and each child is given a probability of classification in each cluster.

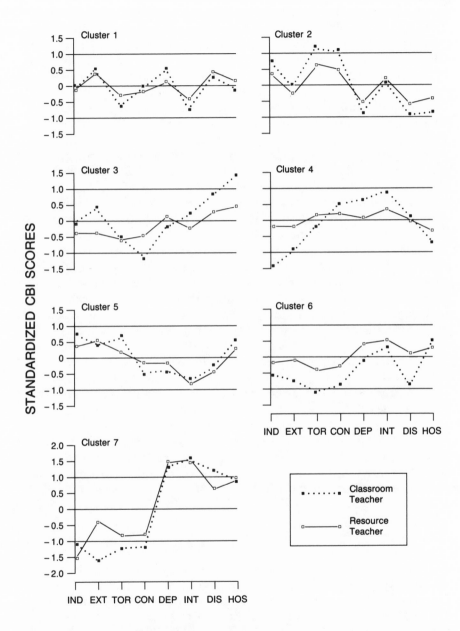

Figure 6.3. Initial ratings by cluster for special education and classroom teachers. (IND = independence; EXT = extroversion; TOR = task orientation; CON = considerateness; DEP = dependence; INT = introversion; DIS = distractibility; HOS = hostility.)

For theoretical and statistical reasons we combined several of the original subtypes into four composite groups that represented the major clinical subdivisions of the sample (Achenbach & Edelbrock, 1981; Schaefer, 1981). Original Clusters 2 and 5 were combined into one subgroup ($n = 15$) that represented normal behavior patterns, and Clusters 3 (conduct problems), 6 (low positive behavior), and 7 (global behavior problems) were combined to form one subgroup ($n = 14$) that represented classroom management problems. The attention deficit ($n = 14$) and withdrawn ($n = 4$) clusters were retained as separate subgroups because of their highly distinctive behavior patterns.

The degree of membership agreement between successive years was assessed by Cohen's kappa, and the stability of original subtype differences in subsequent years was assessed by MANOVA. MANOVAs showed that the original differences among subtypes on CBI scales were maintained in subsequent years. However, there were significant changes in the particular subtype membership of individual children. Twenty-four (55%) children remained in the same subtype in Year 2, and 50% were classified similarly in Year 3. The most stable subgroup (80% for Years 1 to 2, and 60% for Years 1 to 3) were those originally classified as displaying normal behavior patterns. The greatest change individually from Year 1 to Year 3 was from normal patterns to more maladaptive patterns (predominantly attention deficit and problem behavior subtypes); it was more likely for a child who was originally classified as normal to move to a maladaptive subtype (54%) than for a child with a maladaptive pattern originally to move to a more adaptive pattern (11%).

On the other hand, although there was substantial change individually, the original profile patterns derived from classroom teachers' ratings were replicated for the original seven subtypes in subsequent years (see Figure 6.4). In the same vein, special education teachers reproduced similar profile patterns in Years 2 and 3 and continued to show significant agreement with classroom teachers in the description of behavioral subtypes.

Relationship of Subtypes to Academic Progress

Given the results of earlier cross-sectional and longitudinal studies, we were quite surprised to find no significant differences among behavioral subtypes on achievement measures in the first and second grades (Speece et al., 1985). Undaunted, however, we pursued the question longitudinally (McKinney & Speece, 1986). Figure 6.5 shows the longitudinal trends for PIAT achievement scores as a function of the clinical subgroups formed from the original cluster analysis in Year

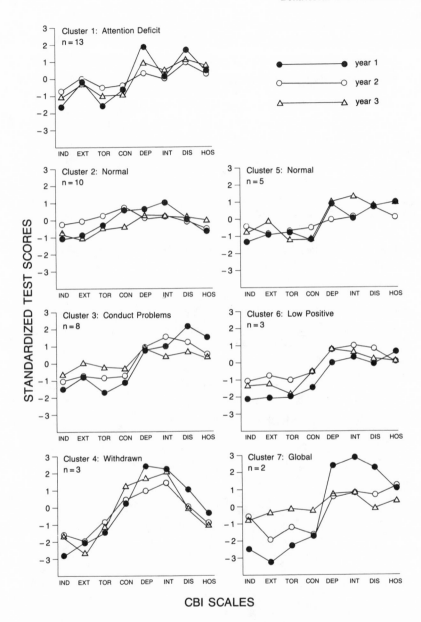

CBI SCALES

Figure 6.4. Longitudinal mean cluster plots for classroom teachers. *Note.* From "Academic Consequences and Longitudinal Stability of Behavioral Subtypes of Learning Disabled Children" by J.D. McKinney & D.L. Speece, 1986, *Journal of Educational Psychology, 78,* p. 370. Copyright 1986 by the *Journal of Educational Psychology.* Reprinted by permission. (IND = independence; EXT = extroversion; TOR = task orientation; CON = considerateness; DEP = dependence; INT = introversion; DIS = distractibility; HOS = hostility.)

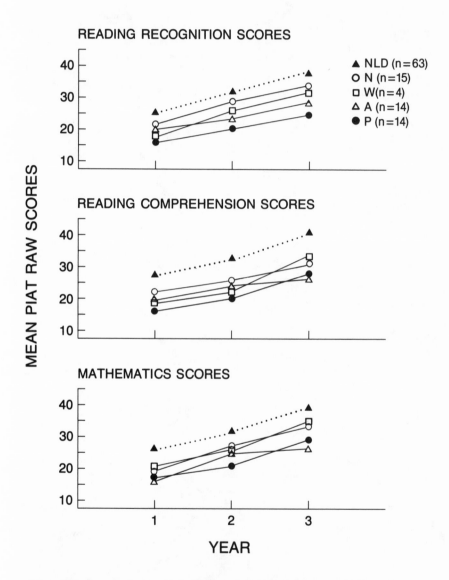

Figure 6.5. Longitudinal trends in Peabody Individual Achievement Test scores by behavioral subtype. *Note.* From "Academic Consequences and Longitudinal Stability of Behavioral Subtypes of Learning Disabled Children" by J.D. McKinney & D.L. Speece, 1986, *Journal of Educational Psychology, 78,* p. 368. Copyright 1986 by the *Journal of Educational Psychology.* Reprinted by permission. (NLD = non-learning-disabled; N = normal LD subtypes; W = withdrawn subtype; A = attentional problems; P = problem behavior.)

1 compared to average achievers. Repeated measures MANOVAs on these data showed significant subgroups × year interactions such that (a) children with LD without significant behavior problems and those with withdrawn behavior displayed a linear pattern similar to that of normal achievers, but continued to show subaverage achievement, and (b) children with LD with attentional and classroom management problems (primarily conduct problems) displayed a declining pattern of progress relative to those in other subgroups and to average achievers.

Thus, while differences in achievement were not evident initially in the first and second grades, children with LD and with some patterns of specific behaviors were at significantly greater risk for poorer academic outcomes than others who presented different patterns of behavior.

CONCLUSIONS

Longitudinal evidence from the Carolina Learning Disabilities Project supports the general conclusion that learning disability is a chronic, seriously handicapping condition that results in persistent underachievement throughout the elementary school period. Further, this pattern of progressive underachievement for the sample as a whole was not easily remediated by the provision of conventional special education services as early as the first and second grades. In general, this prospective evidence confirms other cross-sectional evidence as well as evidence from follow-up studies suggesting that the disparity between most students with LD and same-aged average achievers increases developmentally (Feagans & McKinney, 1981; Kavale, 1988; Werner & Smith, 1977).

On the other hand, this research was successful in identifying a variety of behavioral characteristics that were associated with student academic outcomes developmentally (Feagans & Appelbaum, 1986; McKinney et al., 1985; McKinney & Speece, 1986; Speece et al., 1985). Collectively, results from both cross-sectional and longitudinal studies showed consistent differences between children with LD and normal achievers that persisted over the elementary school years and that produced consistent patterns of correlation with academic outcomes. Also, the pattern of correlation longitudinally was substantially different from that for the comparison group with respect to behavioral characteristics. More importantly, we discovered that children with LD could be classified into more specific subgroups according to their patterns of behavioral strength and weakness, and that those patterns were prognostic of developmental trends in academic progress.

The empirical classification of behavioral subtypes in this research provides a more detailed portrait of behavioral characteristics than that obtained previously with correlational and group comparison research. First, it reveals that not all children with LD exhibit maladaptive behavior patterns. The presence of children with LD in normal subtypes indicates that the underachievement of more than one-third of the sample of children with LD could not be explained solely on the basis of their behavioral characteristics. This has been a common finding in subtype studies that have varied in types of measures, classification procedures, and samples (McKinney, 1988).

Thus, the finding of normal appearing subtypes does not necessarily suggest that the students in this study were misclassified as learning disabled, because multiple factors may be involved in identification and/or account for their underachievement. Consistent findings in this regard have supported the view that learning disabilities reflect multiple syndromes of specific disorders, and indicate the need to develop a theoretically based taxonomy for the classification of specific learning disabilities that allows us to map all the relevant domains of measurement adequately.

One of the more interesting results from the longitudinal study of behavioral subtypes was the clear relationship between children's original subtype membership and individual differences in later outcome in spite of (a) absence of initial differences in achievement among subtypes and (b) significant change in subtype membership over subsequent years. In evaluating the theoretical implications of these findings it is useful to consider (a) those characteristics that were common to maladaptive subtypes, (b) the nature and direction of changes in subtype membership, and (c) the nature of special education services the children received.

First, with respect to the relationship between subtypes and academic progress, although children with attention deficits and problem behaviors showed the most variable subtype membership, the direction of change in subtype membership over the 3-year period of study was toward more maladaptive subtypes rather than toward behaviorally normal subtypes. In general, this pattern of change in subtype membership is consistent with clinical evidence that the social/emotional sequelae associated with repeated failure become more evident among children with LD as they progress through the elementary grades (Lorin, Cowen, & Caldwell, 1974; Routh & Mesibov, 1980), and with prospective studies of at-risk children that show increased risk for conduct and personality disorders for children who are identified as learning disabled in the elementary grades. Thus, while not conclusive, the data on change in subtype membership suggest that attentional and conduct disorders are linked developmentally, and that the presence of either or both in the early elementary grades elevates the risk for poorer achievement later as well as for adjustment problems.

In this regard, it is important that children in the attention deficit and problem behavior subtypes had low task orientation and low independence in common, and that these behaviors have been associated with low academic productivity in the classroom for both general education samples (McKinney et al., 1975) and samples of students with LD (McKinney & Feagans, 1988; McKinney & Speece, 1983). The presence of these behaviors by themselves may be sufficient to establish risk for poorer academic progress early in the elementary period, which is then exacerbated by social/emotional sequelae that develop subsequently.

Finally, the results of these studies should be evaluated in relation to the special education services the children with LD received. Over the first 3 years of the project, children in the longitudinal sample received very similar treatment with respect to the intensity and content of services. Special education was aimed primarily at assistance in basic skills related to the regular classroom curriculum, and was delivered in resource room settings for approximately 1 hour per day for 4 days per week. Although this pattern of special education might be appropriate for some children with LD who do not present significant behavior problems, the results of these studies suggest that more intense and/or behaviorally oriented services may have been more appropriate for many students, and/or that the provision of such services early in the elementary period might have ameliorated the risk associated with poor outcomes for many of these students with unfavorable behavioral characteristics.

REFERENCES

Achenbach, T., & Edelbrock, C. (1981). Behavioral problems and competencies reported by parents of normal and disturbed children aged four through sixteen. *Monographs of the Society for Research in Child Development, 46* (1, Serial No. 188).

Bryan, T. (1974). An observational analysis of classroom behaviors of children with learning disabilities. *Journal of Learning Disabilities, 7,* 35–43.

Bryan, T., & Wheeler, R. (1972). Perception of learning disabled children: The eye of the observer. *Journal of Learning Disabilities, 5,* 484–488.

Cullinan, D., Epstein, M.H., & Denbinski, R.J. (1979). Behavior problems of educationally handicapped normal pupils. *Journal of Abnormal Child Psychology, 7,* 495–502.

Deshler, D. (1978). Psychoeducational aspects of learning disabled adolescents. In L. Mann, L. Goodman, & J.L. Wiederholt (Eds.), *Teaching the learning disabled adolescent.* Boston: Houghton Mifflin.

Dorval, B., McKinney, J.D., & Feagans, L. (1982). Teacher interaction with learning disabled children and average achievers. *Journal of Pediatric Psychology, 17*, 317–330.

Dunn, L.M., & Markwardt, F.C. (1970). *Peabody individual achievement test.* Circle Pines, MN: American Guidance Service.

Farran, D.C., & McKinney, J.D. (1986). *Risk in intellectual and psychosocial development.* New York: Academic Press.

Feagans, L. (1983). Discourse processes in learning disabled children. In J.D. McKinney & L.F. Feagans (Eds.), *Current topics in learning disabilities* (Vol. 1, pp. 87–115). Norwood, NJ: Ablex.

Feagans, L., & Appelbaum, M.I. (1986). Language subtypes and their validation in learning disabled children. *Journal of Educational Psychology, 78,* 373–481.

Feagans, L., & McKinney, J.D. (1980). *Sex differences in learning disabilities.* Unpublished manuscript.

Feagans, L., & McKinney, J.D. (1981). Pattern of exceptionality across domains in learning disabled children. *Journal of Applied Developmental Psychology, 1,* 313–328.

Feagans, L., & Short, E.J. (1984). Developmental differences in the comprehension and production of narratives by reading disabled and normally achieving children. *Child Development, 55,* 1727–1736.

Forman, B.D., & McKinney, J.D. (1975). Teacher perceptions of the classroom behavior of learning disabled and non-learning disabled children. *Proceedings of the National Association of School Psychology, 2,* 285–286.

Forness, S.R., & Esveldt, K.C. (1975). Classroom observation of children with learning and behavior problems. *Journal of Learning Disabilities, 8,* 382–385.

Gottesman, R.L. (1979). Follow-up of learning disabled children. *Learning Disability Quarterly, 2,* 60–69.

Gresham, F.M. (1988). Social competence and motivational characteristics of learning disabled students. In M.C. Wang, H.J. Walberg, & M.C. Reynolds (Eds.), *The handbook of special education: Research and practice* (pp. 283–302). Oxford: Pergamon.

Hoge, R.D., & Luce, S. (1979). Predicting academic achievement from classroom behavior. *Review of Educational Research, 49,* 479–496.

Horn, W.F., O'Donnell, J.P., & Vitulano, L.A. (1983). Long-term follow-up studies of learning disabled persons. *Journal of Learning Disabilities, 16,* 542–555.

Kavale, K.A. (1988). The long-term consequences of learning disabilities. In M.C. Wang, H.J. Walberg, & M.C. Reynolds (Eds.), *The handbook of special education: Research and practice* (pp. 303–344). Oxford: Pergamon.

Lorin, R.P., Cowen, E.L., & Caldwell, R.A. (1974). Problem types of children referred to a school-based mental health program: Identification and outcome. *Journal on Consulting and Clinical Psychology, 47,* 491–496.

Lyon, R. (1983). Subgroups of learning disabled readers: Clinical and empirical identification. In H. Myklebust (Ed.), *Progress in learning disabilities* (Vol. V). New York: Grune & Stratton.

Lyon, R. (1985). Identification and remediation of learning disability subtypes: Preliminary findings. *Learning Disabilities Focus, 1*(1), 21–35.

McKinney, J.D. (1984). The search for subtypes of specific learning disability. *Journal of Learning Disabilities, 17,* 43–50.

McKinney, J.D. (1987). Research on the identification of LD children: Perspectives on changes in educational policy. In S. Vaughn & C. Bos (Eds.), *Issues and future directions in learning disabilities research* (pp. 215–237). San Diego: College-Hill Press.

McKinney, J.D. (1988). Research on conceptually and empirically derived subtypes of specific learning disabilities. In M.C. Wang, H.J. Walberg, & M.C. Reynolds (Eds.), *The handbook of special education: Research and practice.* Oxford: Pergamon.

McKinney, J.D., & Feagans, L. (1980). *Learning disabilities in the classroom.* Chapel Hill, NC: Frank Porter Graham Child Development Center.

McKinney, J.D., & Feagans, L. (1983). Adaptive classroom behavior of learning disabled students. *Journal of Learning Disabilities, 16,* 360–367.

McKinney, J.D., & Feagans, L. (1984). Academic and behavioral characteristics: Longitudinal studies of learning disabled children and average achievers. *Learning Disability Quarterly, 7,* 251–265.

McKinney, J.D., & Feagans, L. (1988). *Academic and behavioral consequences of learning disabilities: Longitudinal follow-up at eleven years of age.* Manuscript submitted for publication.

McKinney, J.D., & Forman, S.G. (1982). Classroom behavior patterns of EMH, LD and EH students. *Journal of School Psychology, 20,* 271–289.

McKinney, J.D., Mason, J., Perkerson, K., & Clifford, M. (1975). Relationship between classroom behavior and achievement. *Journal of Educational Psychology, 67,* 198–203.

McKinney, J.D., McClure, S., & Feagans, L. (1982). Classroom behavior patterns of learning disabled children. *Learning Disability Quarterly, 5,* 45–52.

McKinney, J.D., Short, E.J., & Feagans, L. (1985). Academic consequences of perceptual-linguistic subtypes of learning disabled children. *Learning Disabilities Research, 1*(1), 6–17.

McKinney, J.D., & Speece, D.L. (1983). Classroom behavior and the academic progress of learning disabled students. *Journal of Applied Developmental Psychology, 4,* 149–161.

McKinney, J.D., & Speece, D.L. (1986). Academic consequences and longitudinal stability of behavioral subtypes of learning disabled children. *Journal of Educational Psychology, 78,* 365–372.

Moore, M.G., Haskins, R., & McKinney, J.D. (1980). Classroom behavior patterns of reflective and impulsive children. *Journal of Applied Developmental Psychology, 1,* 59–75.

Oxford, R.B., Morrison, S.B., & McKinney, J.D. (1980). Classroom ecology and off-task behavior of kindergarten students. *The Journal of Classroom Interaction, 15*(1), 34–40.

Porter, J.E., & Rourke, B.P. (1985). Socioemotional functioning of learning disabled children. In B.P. Rourke (Ed.), *Neuropsychology of learning disabilities: Essentials of subtype analysis* (pp. 257–277). New York: Guilford.

Ramey, C.T., & McKinney, J.D. (1981). Education of learning disabled children suspected of minimal brain dysfunction. In P. Black (Ed.), *Brain dysfunction in children: Etiology, diagnosis, and management* (pp. 203–220). New York: Raven.

Richey, D.D., & McKinney, J.D. (1978). Classroom behavior styles of learning disabled children. *Journal of Learning Disabilities, 11,* 38–43.

Rourke, B.P. (1985). *Neuropsychology of learning disabilities: Essentials of subtype analysis.* New York: Guilford Press.

Routh, D.K., & Mesibov, G.B. (1980). Psychological and environmental intervention. In H.F. Rie & E.D. Rie (Eds.), *Handbook of minimal brain dysfunctions* (pp. 618–644). New York: Wiley.

Satz, P., Morris, R., & Fletcher, J.M. (1985). Hypotheses, subtypes and individual differences in dyslexia: Some reflections. In D. Gray & J. Kavanagh (Eds.), *Biobehavioral measures of dyslexia* (pp. 25–40). Parkton, MD: York Press.

Schaefer, E.S. (1981). Development of adaptive behavior: Conceptual models and family correlates. In M. Begab, H. Garber, & H.C. Haywood (Eds.), *Prevention of retarded development in psychosocially disadvantaged children* (pp. 155–179). Austin, TX: PRO-ED.

Schaefer, E.S., Edgerton, M., & Aronson, M. (1977). *Classroom behavior inventory.* Chapel Hill, NC: Frank Porter Graham Child Development Center.

Short, E.J., Feagans, L., McKinney, J.D., & Appelbaum, M.I. (1986). Longitudinal stability of LD subtypes based on age- and IQ-achievement discrepancies. *Learning Disability Quarterly, 9,* 214–225.

Speece, D.L. (1988). *Methodological issues in cluster analysis: How clusters become real.* Paper presented at the International Academy of Research in Learning Disabilities, University of California, Los Angeles.

Speece, D.L., McKinney, J.D., & Appelbaum, M.I. (1985). Classification and validation of behavioral subtypes of learning disabled children. *Journal of Educational Psychology, 77,* 67–77.

Thompson, R.J. (1986). *Behavior problems in children with developmental and learning disabilities* [Monograph No. 3]. Ann Arbor: University of Michigan Press.

Torgesen, J.K. (1975). Problems and prospects in the study of learning disabilities. In E.M. Hetherington (Ed.), *Review of child development research* (Vol. 5). Chicago: University of Chicago Press.

Wechsler, D. (1974). *Wechsler intelligence scale for children–Revised.* New York: Psychological Corp.

Werner, E.E., & Smith, R.S. (1977). *Kauai's children come of age.* Honolulu: University Press of Hawaii.

Wong, B. (1979). The role of theory in learning disabilities research, Part II. A selective review of current theories of learning and reading disabilities. *Journal of Learning Disabilities, 12,* 649–658.

Woodcock, R.W., & Johnson, M.B. (1977). *Woodcock-Johnson psycho-educational battery.* Allen, TX: DLM Teaching Resources.

7. Self-Efficacy and Cognitive Achievement: Implications for Students with Learning Problems

DALE H. SCHUNK

Recent research in various domains has demonstrated that learning is a complex process involving instructional, social, and learner variables (Pintrich, Cross, Kozma, & McKeachie, 1986). The research program that I have been conducting has focused on two related issues. One issue is how social and instructional factors associated with learning contexts affect students' self-perceptions, learning, and motivation. The primary self-perception measure that I have studied is *perceived self-efficacy*, or personal beliefs about one's capabilities to organize and implement actions necessary to attain designated levels of performance (Bandura, 1982). The second issue is how self-efficacy functions as a predictor of achievement behaviors. The subjects in most of these studies have been students who have encountered problems learning academic content. At the outset of these studies, subjects typically display low performance in content area skills and self-efficacy.

The conceptual focus derives from Bandura's (1986) social cognitive learning theory, which views human functioning in terms of reciprocal interactions among behaviors, environmental variables, and cognitions and other personal factors. This reciprocity is well exemplified with perceptions of self-efficacy. Self-efficacy can have diverse effects on achievement behaviors (discussed below). In turn, students' actual performances—their successes and failures at achievement tasks—convey information to them about how well they are learning, which can influence self-efficacy. Self-efficacy is affected by environmental factors, such as when students observe models or receive performance feedback from teachers. Individuals in students' social environments may react to students based on attributes typically associated with them rather than based on what students actually do. Teachers often judge students with learning disabilities (LD) as less capable than nondisabled students and hold lower academic expectations for them, even in content areas where students with LD are performing adequately (Bryan & Bryan, 1983).

One effect of self-efficacy on achievement behaviors involves choice of activities. Students who hold a low sense of efficacy for accomplishing a task may attempt to avoid it, whereas those who believe they are capable should participate more eagerly. Self-efficacy also can affect effort expenditure and persistence. Especially when they encounter difficulties, students who believe that they can perform well ought to work harder and persist longer than those who doubt their capabilities (Bandura, 1982).

Individuals acquire information to assess self-efficacy from their actual performances, vicarious experiences, forms of persuasion, and physiological indexes. In general, one's successes raise efficacy and failures lower it, although once a strong sense of efficacy is developed an occasional failure may not have much impact. In school, students who observe similar peers perform a task may believe that they, too, are capable of performing it. Information acquired vicariously ought to have a weaker influence on efficacy than performance-based information, because vicarious information can be negated by subsequent failure. Students receive persuasive information from teachers (e.g., "You can do this"). Positive feedback can enhance efficacy, but this increase is apt to be short-lived if students' subsequent efforts are poor. Students also derive efficacy information from such physiological indexes as heart rate and sweating. Anxiety symptoms can convey that one lacks the skills to perform well.

I do not wish to imply that self-efficacy is an important variable in all situations. Efficacy appraisal typically does not occur for habitual routines or for tasks requiring skills that are well established (Bandura, 1982). In school, self-efficacy beliefs are likely to be more salient and influential when learning is involved than when students are performing previously learned skills. Even in the former situations, many other variables will affect skill development. Cognitive *abilities* are good predictors of what and how rapidly students learn (Corno & Snow, 1986). *Outcome expectations,* or beliefs concerning the outcomes of one's actions, also are important. Students are generally not motivated to behave in ways that they believe will result in negative outcomes.

Another influence is the *value* students place on outcomes, or how important they believe those outcomes will be for their lives. Students who perceive little value in learning particular content may expend little effort even if they feel efficacious about learning that content (Schunk, in press).

Self-efficacy was originally applied in therapeutic settings with fearful clients (e.g., snake phobics) to help explain their behaviors that are designed to overcome anxiety and cope with threatening activities (Bandura, 1982). Efficacy research has subsequently explored domains such as athletic performances, career choices, and health behaviors. My research has been in educational contexts where students are learning cognitive skills (e.g., mathematics, reading comprehension). Subjects in most of these studies have been elementary or middle school students who previously have experienced learning problems in school and who begin with low skills and perceived efficacy.

Subjects initially are pretested on self-efficacy, skill, and persistence. To assess self-efficacy, testers briefly show subjects samples of the academic content (i.e., math problems, reading passages and questions). For each sample, subjects judge their certainty of solving problems (answering questions) like those shown; thus, subjects judge their capabilities for solving different problems (answering different questions) and not whether they can solve particular problems (answer particular questions). On the skill test, subjects decide whether to solve (answer) each of several problems (questions) and how long to work on them, which provides a measure of persistence. Treatment procedures are subsequently implemented in conjunction with an instructional program on the content area skills. Subjects are posttested on completion of the instructional program.

Recently I have begun to include a measure of *self-efficacy for learning,* or students' beliefs about their capabilities to effectively apply their knowledge and skills to learn academic content. As mentioned earlier, self-efficacy beliefs are likely to be more influential when learning is involved than when students are performing previously learned skills. To assess self-efficacy for learning, testers ask subjects to judge their capability to learn how to solve (answer) different types of problems (questions) rather than their capability for solving (answering) types of problems (questions).

In the following section, I present a self-efficacy model of school learning. Empirical evidence is summarized showing the effects on self-efficacy and achievement behaviors of task engagement (social, instructional) variables. I then discuss evidence for the predictive utility of self-efficacy during cognitive skill learning. The chapter concludes with suggestions for future research and educational implications of the research findings for students with learning problems.

SELF-EFFICACY AND COGNITIVE SKILL LEARNING

Figure 7.1 portrays the hypothesized operation of self-efficacy during cognitive skill learning. I previously have discussed aspects of this model (Schunk, 1984a, 1985b, 1987, in press). It is derived from different theoretical traditions, including social cognitive learning, attribution, and instructional psychology (Bandura, 1986; Corno & Mandinach, 1983; McCombs, 1984; Weiner, 1985; Winne, 1985).

Entry Characteristics

Students differ in *aptitudes* and *prior experiences*. Aptitudes include general abilities, skills, strategies, interests, attitudes, and personality characteristics (Cronbach & Snow, 1977). Educational experiences derive from influences such as prior schools attended, interactions with teachers, and time spent on different subjects. Aptitudes and experiences are related. For example, skilled readers typically perform well on reading tasks, which earns them teacher praise and high grades. In turn, these outcomes may lead students to develop greater interest in reading, which can lead to further skill improvements.

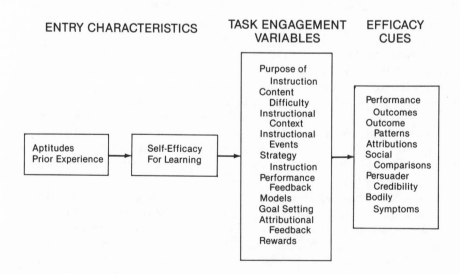

Figure 7.1. Self-efficacy model of cognitive skill learning.

Self-Efficacy for Learning

At the outset of a learning endeavor, we may speak of self-efficacy for learning, acquiring knowledge, developing skills, or mastering material. Aptitudes and prior experiences will affect students' initial beliefs about their learning capabilities. Students who previously have performed well in a content area are apt to believe that they are capable of further learning; students who have experienced difficulties may doubt their capabilities. At the same time, efficacy is not a mere reflection of aptitudes and prior experiences. Using students of high, average, and low mathematical ability, Collins (1982) found students of high and low mathematical self-efficacy within each ability level. Students solved problems and could rework those they missed. Ability was positively related to skillful performance, but regardless of ability level, students with higher efficacy solved more problems correctly and chose to rework more that they missed.

Efficacy Cues

I discuss task engagement variables in the next section. While participating in learning activities, students derive cues that signal how well they are learning and that they use to assess efficacy for continued learning. In turn, higher efficacy for learning enhances motivation and skill acquisition.

Performance outcomes are influential cues. Successes generally raise self-efficacy and failures lower it; however, an occasional failure after many successes may not have much impact, nor should one success after many failures (Schunk, in press). Early learning is often fraught with failures, but the perception of progress can promote efficacy; thus, _outcome patterns_ are important. Self-efficacy may not be aided much if students believe that their progress is slow or that their skills have stabilized at low levels.

Attributions, or perceived causes of successes and failures, influence efficacy in important ways. Achievement outcomes often are attributed to such causes as ability, effort, task difficulty, and luck (Frieze, 1980; Weiner, 1985). Children view effort as the prime cause of outcomes. With development, ability attributions become increasingly important influences on expectancies, and the role of effort declines in importance (Harari & Covington, 1981; Nicholls, 1978). Success achieved with great effort should raise efficacy less than success achieved with minimal effort, because the former implies that skills are not well developed (Bandura, 1982).

Students also derive cues from *social comparisons*. Festinger (1954) hypothesized that, where objective standards of behavior are unclear or unavailable, observers evaluate themselves through comparisons with others, and that the most accurate self-evaluations derive from comparisons with those who are similar in the ability or characteristic being evaluated. Students frequently compare their performances with those of their peers. Students may feel more (less) efficacious when they believe that they are accomplishing more (less) work than most of their peers. Peers also are important models, and observing models is a form of social comparison. Observing similar peers improving their skills can instill a sense of efficacy for learning, whereas observed failures cast doubt on students' capabilities to succeed (Schunk, 1985b). Similarity can be based on perceived competence or on such personal attributes as age, sex, and ethnic background (Rosenthal & Bandura, 1978).

Persuader credibility is important because students may experience higher efficacy when they are told they are capable of learning by a trustworthy source (e.g., the teacher), whereas they may discount the advice of less credible sources. Students also may discount otherwise credible sources if they believe that the sources do not fully understand the nature of the task demands (e.g., difficult for students to comprehend) or the effect of contextual factors (e.g., too many distractions).

Bodily symptoms serve as physiological cues for appraising efficacy. Sweating and trembling may signal that students are not capable of learning. Students who notice that they are reacting in a less agitated fashion to academic tasks may feel more efficacious about learning.

Task Engagement Variables

Task engagement refers to students' cognitive activities (attending, rehearsing, processing, and integrating information), along with their verbalizations and behaviors, that are focused on the academic task at hand (Brophy, 1983; Corno & Mandinach, 1983). Shown in Figure 7.1 are some variables that can impact students while they are engaged in tasks. This list is not exhaustive, but rather is suggestive of influences that seem germane to school learning settings.

The *purpose of instruction* refers to the uses students believe they will make of the material to be learned (Marx, 1983). Students' beliefs about the outcomes of learning can affect self-efficacy. For example, when teachers announce that material will be on a test, students who have performed poorly on tests may experience anxiety, which could lead to low efficacy. Students who previously have earned good grades on term papers may react with high efficacy to the announcement that they will have to write a term paper.

Perceived *content difficulty* is an important task engagement variable. Content that students believe is difficult may lead to a lower sense of self-efficacy for learning than material that students believe is easier to learn. Included here are students' beliefs about the type of cognitive processing required by the content. Students who have trouble processing information required by a task may conclude that they have low ability, and they will feel less efficacious about learning. Salomon (1984) has shown that students perceive learning from TV to be easier than learning from print, hold higher efficacy for learning from TV, and invest less mental effort in learning. For written materials, self-efficacy relates positively to mental effort.

The *instructional context* includes such factors as the setting (physical conditions, distractions), the instructional format (whole class, small group, individualized), materials, and equipment (videotapes, computers). Students' beliefs about how well they learn under these various conditions will affect their efficacy for learning. For example, some students believe that they learn well in an individualized format, whereas others may believe that they derive greater benefits in small groups.

Instructional events include the teacher's explanations, demonstrations, and reteaching, along with students' activities. Teachers who present material in a fashion that students can comprehend are more apt to engender high efficacy than teachers who give disorganized presentations. Use of instructional time also is important. Teachers who provide students with multiple opportunities for task engagement (instruction, practice, review) enhance opportunities to experience success.

Teacher assistance is important. Teachers who provide much assistance to students may improve their skills but do little to raise their self-efficacy for learning, because students may believe that they could not succeed on their own. Also included in this category are teachers' expectations for students' learning, which they often convey to students. Teachers may cue positive (negative) expectations by asserting that students will enjoy (not enjoy) the task and do well (poorly) on it (Brophy, 1983). These statements, coming from a credible judge of student abilities, should impact students' efficacy.

Much research shows that students benefit from training on strategies, or cognitive plans oriented toward improving performance (Baker & Brown, 1984; Paris, Cross, & Lipson, 1984). *Strategy instruction* also can influence self-efficacy. The belief that one understands and can effectively apply a strategy that will enhance achievement can lead to a greater sense of control over learning outcomes, which should promote self-efficacy (Licht & Kistner, 1986; Schunk, in press). At the same time, poor readers often lack conditional knowledge concerning when and why to apply strategies (Myers & Paris, 1978). Providing remedial readers with strategy training and strategy value information, or information that strategy use can improve performance, enhances self-efficacy and skills better than strategy training without value information (Schunk & Rice, 1987).

In learning a strategy, students benefit from verbalizing aloud the component steps while applying them to a task. Overt verbalization can facilitate learning because it directs students' attention to important task features, assists strategy encoding and retention, and helps students work in a systematic fashion (Schunk, 1985b). Verbalization seems especially beneficial for students with learning problems (Borkowski & Cavanaugh, 1979). Schunk and Rice (1984) presented remedial readers in Grades 2 through 4 with instruction in listening comprehension. Half of the children in each grade verbalized strategic steps prior to applying them to questions; the other half received strategy instruction but did not verbalize the steps. Strategy instruction led to higher self-efficacy across grades and promoted performance among third and fourth graders, but not among second graders. Perhaps the demands of verbalization, along with those of the comprehension task itself, were too complex for the youngest subjects. These children may have focused their efforts on the comprehension task, which would have interfered with strategy encoding and retention.

In a follow-up study (Schunk & Rice, 1985), children in Grades 4 and 5 with reading comprehension deficiencies received instruction and practice opportunities. Within each grade, half of the subjects verbalized a strategy prior to applying it. Strategy verbalization led to higher reading comprehension, self-efficacy, and ability attributions across grades. The latter finding suggests that strategy verbalization may enhance self-efficacy through its effect on ability attributions.

Schunk and Cox (1986) compared the effects of different forms of verbalization among students with LD during mathematics instruction. Continuously verbalizing a strategy while solving problems led to higher self-efficacy and skill compared with discontinued verbalization or no verbalization. It is possible that, when instructed to no longer verbalize aloud, discontinued verbalization students had difficulty internalizing the strategy and did not use covert instructions to regulate their performances. A fading treatment, such as that included in self-instructional training (Meichenbaum, 1977), can promote strategy internalization.

Performance feedback (e.g., "You're doing much better") can signal that students are making progress in learning, which raises self-efficacy. Teacher feedback is less important when students can derive their own feedback, such as by checking answers. Students benefit from feedback in situations where progress in learning is unclear.

Exposure to *models* is an important task engagement variable. In school, students observe diverse adult and peer models. Perceived similarity of observers and models is a cue used to assess self-efficacy. Models who are similar or slightly higher in competence provide the best information. Students who observe a similar peer learn a task are apt to believe that they can learn as well (Schunk, 1985b). Peer models may exert more beneficial effects on self-efficacy than teacher models, especially among students with learning problems who doubt that they are capable of attaining the teacher's level of competence.

One way to enhance perceived similarity is to use multiple models, which increase the probability that observers will perceive themselves as similar to at least one of the models (Thelen, Fry, Fehrenbach, & Frautschi, 1979). Another way is to use coping rather than mastery models. Coping models initially demonstrate the typical fears and deficiencies of observers but gradually improve their performances and gain self-confidence, whereas mastery models demonstrate faultless performance from the outset (Kazdin, 1978). Coping models illustrate how determined effort and positive thoughts can overcome difficulties.

These ideas were tested with elementary school children who had experienced learning problems in mathematics (Schunk & Hanson, 1985; Schunk, Hanson, & Cox, 1987). Children observed videotapes portraying an adult teacher and one or more peer (student) models. The teacher repeatedly provided instruction, after which the models solved problems. Some subjects observed peer mastery models, who easily grasped the operations, solved all problems correctly, and verbalized positive achievement beliefs reflecting high self-efficacy and ability, low task difficulty, and positive attitudes. Others observed coping models, who initially made errors and verbalized negative achievement beliefs but gradually began to verbalize coping statements (e.g., "I'll have to work hard on this one") and became more skillful. Eventually the coping models' problem-solving behaviors and verbalizations matched those of the mastery models. Other children observed only a teacher model or did not observe videotapes.

Observing peer models enhanced self-efficacy for learning, along with posttest self-efficacy and skillful performance, more than observing a teacher model or not observing a model. Schunk and Hanson (1985) found no differential effects of coping and mastery models on children's self-efficacy and skills. Subjects had experienced prior successes with the experimental content (subtraction of whole numbers), and may have drawn on those experiences and focused more on what the models had in common (task success) than on their differences (rate of learning, number of errors, types of verbalization). In contrast, the

Schunk et al. (1987) subjects had few, if any, prior successes with the content (addition and subtraction of fractions). In this study, coping models enhanced achievement outcomes more than observing mastery models, and multiple models—coping or mastery—promoted achievement outcomes as well as a single coping model and better than a single mastery model. Children who observed single models judged themselves more similar in competence to coping models than to mastery models. The benefits of multiple models did not depend on perceived similarity in competence. Similarity in competence may be a more important source of efficacy information when children are exposed to a single model and have fewer modeled cues to use in judging self-efficacy.

Goal setting involves comparing one's present performance against a standard. When students pursue a goal, they may experience heightened self-efficacy for attaining it as they observe their goal progress. A sense of learning efficacy helps sustain task motivation. Goals exert their effects through their properties: specificity, difficulty level, proximity (Bandura & Cervone, 1983; Locke, Shaw, Saari, & Latham, 1981). Goals that incorporate specific performance standards are more likely to raise learning efficacy because progress toward an explicit goal is easier to gauge. General goals (e.g., "Do your best") do not enhance motivation. In the context of an instructional program, Schunk (1985a) found that specific performance goals—whether self-set or set by teachers—enhanced mathematics achievement and self-efficacy more than no goals in students with LD.

Goal difficulty refers to the level of task proficiency required as assessed against a standard. Although students initially may doubt their capabilities to attain goals they believe are difficult, working toward difficult goals can build a strong sense of efficacy, because difficult goals offer more information about learning capabilities than easier goals.

Goals also are distinguished by how far they project into the future. Proximal goals, which are close at hand, result in greater motivation than more distant goals. As students observe their progress toward a proximal goal, they are apt to believe that they are capable of further learning. During an instructional program, Schunk (1983b) found that providing students with proximal goals enhanced their mathematical self-efficacy more than no goals. Bandura and Schunk (1981) found that, compared with distal or no goals, proximal goals heightened children's task motivation and led to the highest mathematical self-efficacy, interest, and skillful performance. Distal goals resulted in no benefits over those obtained from receiving the instructional program.

Attributional feedback, which links students' successes and failures with one or more causes, is a persuasive source of efficacy information. Young children stress the role of effort. Although ability information becomes more important with development (Nicholls, 1978), effort feedback can motivate students of different ages. Being told that one can achieve better results through harder work (i.e., effort feedback for prior difficulties) can motivate one to do so and convey that one possesses the necessary capability to succeed (Andrews & Debus, 1978; Dweck, 1975). Providing effort feedback for prior successes supports students' perceptions of their progress in learning, sustains motivation, and increases efficacy for continued learning (Schunk, 1985b). Effort feedback may be especially useful for students with learning problems, who often place insufficient emphasis on the role of effort in achievement contexts (Torgesen & Licht, 1983).

Teacher praise can affect self-efficacy for learning, because praise conveys how the teacher views student abilities (Weiner, Graham, Taylor, & Meyer, 1983). Especially when students believe that a task is easy, praise combined with effort information (e.g., "That's good. You've been working hard") signals low ability. Students who believe that the teacher does not expect much of them are apt to doubt their capabilities.

The timing of attributional feedback also is important. Early task successes constitute a prominent cue used to formulate ability attributions (Weiner, 1974). Feedback that links students' early successes with ability (e.g., "That's correct. You're really good at this") should enhance learning efficacy. Many times, however, effort feedback for early successes may be more credible, because when students lack skills they realistically have to expend effort to succeed. As students develop skills, switching to ability feedback may better enhance self-efficacy.

These ideas have been tested in several studies (Schunk, 1982, 1983a, 1984b; Schunk & Cox, 1986). Schunk (1982) found that linking children's prior achievements with effort (e.g., "You've been working hard") led to higher task motivation, self-efficacy, and subtraction skill, compared with linking their future achievement with effort ("You need to work hard") or not providing effort feedback. Schunk (1983a) showed that ability feedback for prior successes ("You're good at this") enhanced self-efficacy and skill better than effort feedback of ability-plus-effort (combined) feedback. The latter subjects judged their effort expenditure during the instructional program greater than ability-only students. Children in the combined condition may have discounted some ability information in favor of effort.

To investigate sequence effects, Schunk (1984b) periodically provided one group of children with ability feedback, a second group with effort feedback, and a third group with ability feedback during the first half of training and effort feedback during the second half. This latter sequence was reversed for a fourth condition. Providing ability feedback for early success, regardless of whether it was continued, led to higher ability attributions and posttest self-efficacy and skill, compared with providing effort feedback for early success.

In the Schunk and Cox (1986) study, students received effort feedback during the first half of the instructional program, effort feedback during the second half, or no effort feedback. Each type of feedback promoted self-efficacy and skillful performance better than no feedback; feedback during the first half of training enhanced students' effort attributions. Given students' learning disabilities, effort feedback for early or later successes may have seemed credible, because the students realistically had to expend effort to succeed. Over time, effort feedback could actually lower efficacy, because as students become more skillful they might wonder why they still have to work hard to succeed.

Rewards can promote task performance (Lepper & Greene, 1978) and can enhance self-efficacy when they are tied to students' actual accomplishments. Telling students that they can earn rewards based on what they accomplish can instill a sense of efficacy for learning. As students work at a task and note their progress, this sense of efficacy is validated. Receipt of the reward further validates self-efficacy, because it symbolizes progress. When rewards are not tied to actual performance, they actually may convey negative efficacy information; students might infer that they are not expected to learn much because they do not possess the requisite capability. In the context of a long division instructional program, Schunk (1983c) found that performance-contingent rewards led to more rapid problem solving, as well as higher skill and self-efficacy, compared with task-contingent rewards and unexpected rewards. Offering rewards for participation (task-contingent) led to no benefits over those due to receiving instruction.

Predictive Utility of Self-Efficacy

The predictive utility of self-efficacy for learning can be determined by relating this measure to the number of problems that children complete during the independent practice portions of instructional sessions. Significant and positive correlations have been obtained (range of $rs = .33$ to $.42$). More rapid problem solving has not been attained at the expense of accuracy. Similar correlations have been obtained using the proportion of problems solved correctly. Self-efficacy for learning also relates positively to posttest self-efficacy and skill (range of $rs = .46$ to $.90$).

The predictive utility of pretest efficacy is often inadequate because subjects lack skills and judge efficacy low. In contrast, there is a greater variability in posttest measures of efficacy and skill. Studies in different domains have yielded significant and positive correlations between posttest efficacy and skill (range of $rs = .27$ to .84).

Multiple regression has been used to determine the percentage of variability in skillful performance accounted for by self-efficacy. These analyses show that perceived efficacy accounts for a significant increment in the variability in posttest skill; R^2 values range from .17 to .24. Schunk (1981) employed path analysis to test how well a causal model of achievement reproduced the original correlation matrix comprising instructional treatment, self-efficacy, persistence, and skill. The most parsimonious model that reproduced the data showed that treatment exerted both a direct effect on skill and an indirect effect through persistence and efficacy, that the effect of treatment on persistence operated indirectly through efficacy, and that efficacy influenced skill and persistence.

FUTURE DIRECTIONS

Research is needed on whether task engagement variables operate differently during various phases of instruction. Students engaged in learning activities may initially perceive material as difficult. These perceptions will change as they receive additional instruction and practice. Perceived content difficulty may be a better predictor of self-efficacy during the later stages of learning.

Further exploration of motivational indexes is needed. Choice of activities is not a good motivational index because students typically do not choose whether to participate in learning activities (Brophy, 1983). Choice is meaningful only under a limited set of conditions (e.g., free time).

High efficacy will not necessarily lead to greater persistence. Students may persist at tasks because of high efficacy for learning but also because teachers keep them working on the tasks. As skills develop, self-efficacy might bear a negative, rather than a positive, relationship to persistence; students should not have to persist as long to solve problems correctly or answer questions. The studies summarized in the preceding section yielded persistence-efficacy correlations ranging from $+.30$ to $-.29$. Where skill learning is involved, cognitive effort seems to be a more appropriate motivational index (Corno & Mandinach, 1983). Research might explore students' cognitive efforts during instruction and relate these to self-efficacy for learning.

Developmental research is needed to explore the cues that students derive from task variables and how students cognitively process these cues to form efficacy beliefs. For example, young children's social comparisons focus on the overt performances of their peers. As children acquire a conception of underlying abilities, the basis for perceived similarity shifts from tangible outcomes to underlying abilities. Whom children use as the basis for social comparisons is an important question. Many students with learning problems spend part of the school day in resource rooms and the remainder in regular classes, and employ both groups for social comparisons. Academically handicapped students may perceive their abilities higher when they compare themselves with other handicapped peers than when they compare themselves with regular class students (Coleman, 1983; Strang, Smith, & Rogers, 1978).

Research could examine the judgment-making process among students with learning problems. To accurately judge efficacy requires that one distinguish successes from failures. Judging efficacy in cognitive skill learning contexts often is complex. Students may learn only some of the component subskills of a task. Being unaware of the full range of task demands can lead to efficacy misjudgment. In mathematics, students often employ *buggy algorithms,* or erroneous strategies that result in problem solutions (Brown & Burton, 1978). Because buggy algorithms produce solutions, employing them may lead to a false sense of competence. Similarly, students who solve problems correctly but are unsure whether their answers are correct may not feel more efficacious.

Students with learning problems often enter a cycle in which school failure and ability self-doubts influence each other (Licht & Kistner, 1986). Yet not all students with learning problems enter this cycle; some feel confident about learning in spite of repeated difficulties. We might examine the judgment-making processes of these latter students. Do they employ buggy algorithms, or are they aware of their learning problems but expect that such factors as heightened task attention and effort expenditure will produce better results in the future?

Another area to address is maintenance and transfer of efficacy beliefs. Many educational interventions are brief—3 weeks or less. Especially with complex cognitive skills, increases in efficacy brought about by relatively short interventions may not prove durable over time or transfer to classroom (nonexperimental) settings. Strategy training research, for example, shows that students often do not maintain their use of strategies or transfer them outside of the experimental context (Borkowski & Cavanaugh, 1979). These problems arise in part because students believe that such factors as effort expended and time available are more important influences on their achievement than is their use of strategies (Fabricius & Hagen, 1984). Maintenance and transfer should be facilitated by including multiple tasks in lengthier interventions. By working with teachers, researchers can study how self-efficacy beliefs change over the course of a semester or school year. A future research agenda might well include teachers as active research collaborators.

EDUCATIONAL IMPLICATIONS

The procedures discussed in this article can be implemented by teachers. For example, the comprehension procedures were applied to children's regular reading groups (Schunk & Rice, 1984, 1985, 1987). Teaching students to use a comprehension strategy by having them verbalize steps is easily implemented in small group reading instruction, and fits well with the suggestion by researchers to teach strategies to students, especially those with learning problems (Borkowski & Cavanaugh, 1979; Brown, Palincsar, & Armbruster, 1984; Paris et al., 1984; Raphael & McKinney, 1983).

Teachers' instructional presentations can include information designed to affect students' self-efficacy. Brophy (1983) discusses various types of task presentation statements made by elementary teachers. Two contrasting types are positive expectations for students (e.g., "I know that you'll learn this") and negative expectations ("Some of you might find this hard"). These types of statements are forms of persuasive information and, given that they are uttered by a credible source, can have important effects on students' efficacy for learning. Although students' subsequent efforts will validate or refute this efficacy information, teachers can have an important impact on students' initial learning beliefs.

Performance and attributional feedback can be applied to seatwork activities. Performance feedback that signals progress in learning validates students' beliefs that they are acquiring skills, and can enhance motivation for further learning. It is important that attributional feedback be viewed as credible by students. Effort feedback for success at a task that students believe is easy may lead them to wonder whether the teacher thinks they are low in ability (Weiner et al., 1983). Similarly, students may discount ability feedback after they have had to struggle to succeed.

Goal setting can be incorporated in various ways. Teachers have lesson goals for students. Contingency contracts specify learning or performance goals. Goal-setting conferences, in which teachers meet periodically with students to discuss their goal attainment and to set new goals, enhance achievement and capability self-evaluations (Gaa,

1973). Short-term goals are maximally motivating with young children, and may be especially beneficial for students with learning problems because they provide concrete standards against which to gauge progress.

Peer models seem especially useful for children with learning problems who may doubt their learning capabilities. Observation of an adult teacher flawlessly demonstrating cognitive skills may teach students skills but not help build efficacy for learning. Such students may view the teacher as possessing a level of competence that they are unlikely to attain. Observing similar peers successfully perform a task can raise self-efficacy in students because they are apt to believe that if the peers can learn, they can also improve their skills.

Teachers often apply these ideas by selecting one or more students to demonstrate a skill to other class members. The typical practice is to choose peers who master skills readily—mastery models. Among students with learning problems, other students who have learning problems, but who have mastered skills, may make better models. Peers also could model such coping behaviors as increased concentration and hard work. While students are engaged in seatwork, teachers can provide social comparative information (e.g., "See how well Kevin is doing? I'm sure that you can do just as well"). Teachers need to insure that learners will view the comparative performances as attainable; judicious selection of referent students is necessary.

Peers also can be used to enhance observers' self-efficacy in small groups. Successful groups in which each member is responsible for some aspect of the task and in which members share rewards based on their collective performance can reduce negative, ability-related social comparisons (Ames, 1984). Teachers need to select tasks carefully, because unsuccessful groups will not raise efficacy.

Strain and his colleagues have successfully used peers as social skill trainers with withdrawn children (Strain, Kerr, & Ragland, 1981). Peers are trained to initiate social contacts with verbal signals and motor responses. Such initiations increase withdrawn children's subsequent social initiations, and gains often generalize to classrooms. A less formal application involves pairing a socially competent peer with a less competent child to work on a task. The opportunity for social interaction within the dyad can help to promote the social skills of the less competent child (Mize, Ladd, & Price, 1985).

The use of peers as instructional agents has most commonly occurred in tutoring programs. Despite some methodological problems in studies, tutoring can lead to academic gains by tutor and tutee (Feldman, Devin-Sheehan, & Allen, 1976). Peer instructors also are helpful where their teaching strategies fit well with learners' capabilities or the skills being taught. Adult teachers typically employ more verbal instruction and relate information to be learned to other material, whereas peer teachers tend to use nonverbal demonstrations and link instruction to specific items (Ellis & Rogoff, 1982). Peer instruction seems beneficial for students with learning problems and for other learners who may not process verbal material particularly well.

REFERENCES

Ames, C. (1984). Competitive, cooperative, and individualistic goal structures: A cognitive-motivational analysis. In R. Ames & C. Ames (Eds.), *Research on motivation in education: Student motivation* (Vol. 1, pp. 177–207). Orlando, FL: Academic Press.

Andrews, G.R., & Debus, R.L. (1978). Persistence and the causal perception of failure: Modifying cognitive attributions. *Journal of Educational Psychology, 70,* 154–166.

Baker, L., & Brown, A.L. (1984). Metacognitive skills and reading. In P.D. Pearson (Ed.), *Handbook of reading research* (pp. 353–394). New York: Longman.

Bandura, A. (1982). Self-efficacy mechanism in human agency. *American Psychologist, 37,* 122–147.

Bandura, A. (1986). *Social foundations of thought and action: A social cognitive theory.* Englewood Cliffs, NJ: Prentice-Hall.

Bandura, A., & Cervone, D. (1983). Self-evaluative and self-efficacy mechanisms governing the motivational effects of goal systems. *Journal of Personality and Social Psychology, 45,* 1017–1028.

Bandura, A., & Schunk, D.H. (1981). Cultivating competence, self-efficacy, and intrinsic interest through proximal self-motivation. *Journal of Personality and Social Psychology, 41,* 586–598.

Borkowski, J.G., & Cavanaugh, J.C. (1979). Maintenance and generalization of skills and strategies by the retarded. In N.R. Ellis (Ed.), *Handbook of mental deficiency, psychological theory and research* (2nd ed., pp. 569–617). Hillsdale, NJ: Erlbaum.

Brophy, J. (1983). Conceptualizing student motivation. *Educational Psychologist, 18,* 200–215.

Brown, J.S., & Burton, R.R. (1978). Diagnostic models for procedural bugs in basic mathematical skills. *Cognitive Science, 2,* 155–192.

Brown, A.L., Palincsar, A.S., & Armbruster, B.B. (1984). Instructing comprehension-fostering activities in interactive learning situations. In H. Mandl, N.L. Stein, & T. Trabasso (Eds.), *Learning and comprehension of text* (pp. 255–286). Hillsdale, NJ: Erlbaum.

Bryan, J.H., & Bryan, T.H. (1983). The social life of the learning disabled youngster. In J.D. McKinney & L. Feagans (Eds.), *Current topics in learning disabilities* (Vol. 1, pp. 57–85). Norwood, NJ: Ablex.

Coleman, J.M. (1983). Self-concept and the mildly handicapped: The role of social comparisons. *The Journal of Special Education, 17,* 37–45.

Collins, J. (1982, March). *Self-efficacy and ability in achievement behavior.* Paper presented at the meeting of the American Educational Research Association, New York.

Corno, L., & Mandinach, E.B. (1983). The role of cognitive engagement in classroom learning and motivation. *Educational Psychologist, 18,* 88–108.

Corno, L., & Snow, R.E. (1986). Adapting teaching to individual differences among learners. In M.C. Wittrock (Ed.), *Handbook of research on teaching* (3rd ed., pp. 605–629). New York: Macmillan.

Cronbach, L.J., & Snow, R.E. (1977). *Aptitudes and instructional methods.* New York: Irvington.

Dweck, C.S. (1975). The role of expectations and attributions in the alleviation of learned helplessness. *Journal of Personality and Social Psychology, 31,* 674–685.

Ellis, S., & Rogoff, B. (1982). The strategies and efficacy of child versus adult teachers. *Child Development, 53,* 730–735.

Fabricius, W.V., & Hagen, J.W. (1984). Use of causal attributions about recall performance to assess metamemory and predict strategic memory behavior in young children. *Developmental Psychology, 20,* 975–987.

Feldman, R.S., Devin-Sheehan, L., & Allen, V.L. (1976). Children tutoring children: A critical review of research. In V.L. Allen (Ed.), *Children as teachers: Theory and research on tutoring* (pp. 235–252). New York: Academic Press.

Festinger, L. (1954). A theory of social comparison processes. *Human Relations, 7,* 117–140.

Frieze, I.H. (1980). Beliefs about success and failure in the classroom. In J.H. McMillan (Ed.), *The social psychology of school learning* (pp. 39–78). New York: Academic Press.

Gaa, J.P. (1973). Effects of individual goal-setting conferences on achievement, attitudes, and goal-setting behavior. *Journal of Experimental Education, 42,* 22–28.

Harari, O., & Covington, M.V. (1981). Reactions to achievement behavior from a teacher and student perspective: A developmental analysis. *American Educational Research Journal, 18,* 15–28.

Kazdin, A.E. (1978). Covert modeling: The therapeutic application of imagined rehearsal. In J.L. Singer & K.S. Pope (Eds.), *The power of human imagination: New methods in psychotherapy* (pp. 255–278). New York: Plenum.

Lepper, M.R., & Greene, D. (1978). *The hidden costs of reward: New perspectives on the psychology of human motivation.* Hillsdale, NJ: Erlbaum.

Licht, B.G., & Kistner, J.A. (1986). Motivational problems of learning-disabled children: Individual differences and their implications for treatment. In J.K. Torgesen & B.W.L. Wong (Eds.), *Psychological and educational perspectives on learning disabilities* (pp. 225–255). Orlando, FL: Academic Press.

Locke, E.A., Shaw, K.N., Saari, L.M., & Latham, G.P. (1981). Goal setting and task performance: 1969–1980. *Psychological Bulletin, 90,* 125–152.

Marx, R.W. (1983). Student perception in classrooms. *Educational Psychologist, 18,* 145–164.

McCombs, B.L. (1984). Processes and skills underlying continuing intrinsic motivation to learn: Toward a definition of motivational skills training interventions. *Educational Psychologist, 19,* 199–218.

Meichenbaum, D. (1977). *Cognitive behavior modification: An integrative approach.* New York: Plenum Press.

Mize, J., Ladd, G.W., & Price, J.M. (1985). Promoting positive peer relations with young children: Rationales and strategies. *Child Care Quarterly, 14,* 221–237.

Myers, M., & Paris, S.G. 1978). Children's metacognitive knowledge about reading. *Journal of Educational Psychology, 70,* 680–690.

Nicholls, J.G. (1978). The development of the concepts of effort and ability, perception of academic attainment, and the understanding that difficult tasks require more ability. *Child Development, 49,* 800–814.

Paris, S.G., Cross, D.R., & Lipson, M.Y. (1984). Informed strategies for learning: A program to improve children's reading awareness and comprehension. *Journal of Educational Psychology, 76,* 1239–1252.

Pintrich, P.R., Cross, D.R., Kozma, R.B., & McKeachie, W.J. (1986). Instructional psychology. *Annual Review of Psychology, 37,* 611–651.

Raphael, T.E., & McKinney, J. (1983). An examination of fifth- and eighth-grade children's question-answering behavior: An instructional study in metacognition. *Journal of Reading Behavior, 15,* 67–86.

Rosenthal, T.L., & Bandura, A. (1978). Psychological modeling: Theory and practice. In S.L. Garfield & A.E. Bergin (Eds.), *Handbook of psychotherapy and behavior change: An empirical analysis* (2nd ed., pp. 621–658). New York: Wiley.

Salomon, G. (1984). Television is "easy" and print is "tough": The differential investment of mental effort in learning as a function of perceptions and attributions. *Journal of Educational Psychology, 76,* 647–658.

Schunk, D.H. (1981). Modeling and attributional effects on children's achievement: A self-efficacy analysis. *Journal of Educational Psychology, 73,* 93–105.

Schunk, D.H. (1982). Effects of effort attributional feedback on children's perceived self-efficacy and achievement. *Journal of Educational Psychology, 74,* 548–556.

Schunk, D.H. (1983a). Ability versus effort attributional feedback: Differential effects on self-efficacy and achievement. *Journal of Educational Psychology, 75,* 848–856.

Schunk, D.H. (1983b). Developing children's self-efficacy and skills: The roles of social comparative information and goal setting. *Contemporary Educational Psychology, 8,* 76–86.

Schunk, D.H. (1983c). Reward contingencies and the development of children's skills and self-efficacy. *Journal of Educational Psychology, 75,* 511–518.

Schunk, D.H. (1984a). Self-efficacy perspective on achievement behavior. *Educational Psychologist, 19,* 48–58.

Schunk, D.H. (1984b). Sequential attributional feedback and children's achievement behaviors. *Journal of Educational Psychology, 76,* 1159–1169.

Schunk, D.H. (1985a). Participation in goal setting: Effects on self-efficacy and skills of learning disabled children. *The Journal of Special Education, 19,* 307–317.

Schunk, D.H. (1985b). Self-efficacy and classroom learning. *Psychology in the Schools, 22,* 208–223.

Schunk, D.H. (1987). Self-efficacy and motivated learning. In N. Hastings & J. Schwieso (Eds.), *New directions in educational psychology: 2. Behaviour and motivation in the classroom* (pp. 233–251). London: The Falmer Press.

Schunk, D.H. (in press). Self-efficacy and performance. In R.E. Ames & C. Ames (Eds.), *Research on motivation in education* (Vol. 3). Orlando, FL: Academic Press.

Schunk, D.H., & Cox, P.D. (1986). Strategy training and attributional feedback with learning disabled students. *Journal of Educational Psychology, 78,* 201–209.

Schunk, D.H., & Hanson, A.R. (1985). Peer models: Influence on children's self-efficacy and achievement. *Journal of Educational Psychology, 77,* 313–322.

Schunk, D.H., Hanson, A.R., & Cox, P.D. (1987). Peer model attributes and children's achievement behaviors. *Journal of Educational Psychology, 79,* 54–61.

Schunk, D.H., & Rice, J.M. (1984). Strategy self-verbalization during remedial listening comprehension instruction. *Journal of Experimental Education, 53,* 49–54.

Schunk, D.H., & Rice, J.M. (1985). Verbalization of comprehension strategies: Effects on children's achievement outcomes. *Human Learning, 4,* 1–10.

Schunk, D.H., & Rice, J.M. (1987). Enhancing comprehension skill and self-efficacy with strategy value information. *Journal of Reading Behavior, 19,* 285–302.

Strain, P.S., Kerr, M.M., & Ragland, E.U. (1981). The use of peer social initiations in the treatment of social withdrawal. In P.S. Strain (Ed.), *The utilization of classroom peers as behavior change agents* (pp. 101–128). New York: Plenum Press.

Strang, L., Smith, M.D., & Rogers, C.M. (1978). Social comparison, multiple reference groups, and the self-concepts of academically handicapped children before and after mainstreaming. *Journal of Educational Psychology, 70,* 487–497.

Thelen, M.H., Fry, R.A., Fehrenbach, P.A., & Frautschi, N.M. (1979). Therapeutic videotape and film modeling: A review. *Psychological Bulletin, 86,* 701–720.

Torgesen, J.K., & Licht, B.G. (1983). The learning disabled child as an inactive learner: Retrospect and prospects. In J.D. McKinney & L. Feagans (Eds.), *Current topics in learning disabilities* (Vol. 1, pp. 3–31). Norwood, NJ: Ablex.

Weiner, B. (1974). An attributional interpretation of expectancy-value theory. In B. Weiner (Ed.), *Cognitive views of human motivation* (pp. 51–69). New York: Academic Press.

Weiner, B. (1985). An attributional theory of achievement motivation and emotion. *Psychological Review, 92,* 548–573.

Weiner, B., Graham, S., Taylor, S.E., & Meyer, W. (1983). Social cognition in the classroom. *Educational Psychologist, 18,* 109–124.

Winne, P.H. (1985). Cognitive processing in the classroom. In T. Husen & T.N. Postlethwaite (Eds.), *The international encyclopedia of education* (Vol. 2, pp. 795–808). Oxford: Pergamon.

8. On Learning ... More or Less: A Knowledge × Process × Context View of Learning Disabilities

STEPHEN J. CECI AND JACQUELYN G. BAKER

When Joe Torgesen invited us to write this chapter, he suggested that we describe our past and present research and avoid attempting a broader synthesis. While we intend to do just this, we also want to do something more as well. We want to describe the direction our current work has taken because it represents a shift from our past research. Later, we will give a bird's-eye glimpse of this new work, but for now we want to alert the reader to the fact that our more recent work, while not being discontinuous from our earlier work, is aimed at a broader, some might even say expansive, question—namely, the contextual, educational, and biological forces that co-mingle to shape cognitive performance. We shall have more to say about this later. But for now, we wish to suggest that this orientation will take us a bit further toward dealing with the dissatisfactions that recently were espoused by respondents to Adelman and Taylor's (1986) survey, as it addresses the problem of the nature of learning disabilities from a normative-individual differences perspective that considers the normal course of developmental changes in processing and in the structure of children's knowledge.

Ten years ago, the first author was drawn to the educational implications of work on memory development, especially semantic memory development. Colleagues Stephen Lea and Maureen Ringstrom and we studied the manner in which children with learning disabilities coded language-based events into memory, vis-à-vis their nondisabled peers (non-LDs). Learning disabilities (LD) was defined on the basis of an IQ-achievement disparity (as opposed to a regression equation approach that has been used in subsequent work), in addition to the diagnosis by the school's multidisciplinary team. As this research predated modern subgrouping studies that employ cluster analysis of galaxies of cognitive measures, it was begun rather simply by classifying children with LD into one of four groups, based solely on their auditory and visual short-term memory ability: (1) children with good visual memory but poor auditory memory (+VIS, −AUD), (2) children with poor visual memory but good auditory memory (−VIS, +AUD), (3) children with poor visual *and* poor auditory memory (−VIS, −AUD), and finally, (4) children with good visual *and* good auditory memory (+VIS, +AUD). In all of our studies, we also included a group of non-LD agemates, some of whom had comparable IQs and others who had lower IQs.

After exposing children to a series of visual and auditory stimuli, we gave them free and cued recall tests. Here, we will focus on the results of the cued recall test because they lead most directly to the studies that we will describe later. Semantic and nonsemantic cues were provided to the children, the former being a stimulus category label and the latter being, in the case of the visually presented stimuli, a stimulus color as well as the spatial location in which it had appeared, and in the case of auditorily presented stimuli, the stimulus acoustic (gender of voice) and phonetic (rhyming) characteristics.

You can see from the results in Figures 8.1a and 8.1b that systematic differences emerged among these four groups of children with LD. Two things struck us immediately. First, nonsemantic cues appeared to work equally well for all groups, except those with poor visual *and* poor auditory memories. This group of children was by far the most severely disabled in our sample in terms of both their school performance and their IQs. Although nonsemantic cues were equally effective across groups, they were not as effective as semantic cues in prompting a child's recollection of the stimuli. Specifically, semantic cues yielded approximately 30% more recall than did nonsemantic cues. Second, a memory impairment in a specific modality was often associated with a reduction in semantic processing in that modality but not with a reduction in nonsemantic processing. Figure 8.1a, for example, shows that children with poor short-term auditory memories were especially poor at using semantic cues to retrieve stimuli that had been presented auditorily. Figure 8.1b shows that children with poor short-term *visual* memories were especially impaired at using semantic cues to retrieve stimuli that had been presented visually. (Not

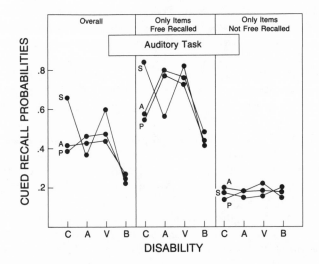

Figure 8.1a. Probability (valence) of correctly recalling an item in response to (S) semantic (category labels), (A) acoustic (gender of speaker's voice), and (P) phonetic (rhymes) cues. Along the abscissa, C = control group (no learning disability), A = group with impaired auditory memory, V = group with impaired visual memory, and B = group with impaired auditory *and* visual memory.

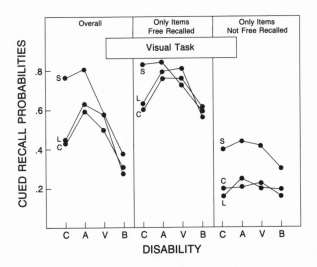

Figure 8.1b. Probability (valence) of correctly recalling an item in response to (S) semantic (category labels), (L) location, and (C) color cues. Along the abscissa, C = control group (no learning disability), A = group with impaired auditory memory, V = group with impaired visual memory, and B = group with impaired auditory *and* visual memory.

shown are the results of cross-modal cuing, in which children were presented items in one modality but cued in a different one. Those results were congruent with the interpretation of a semantic deficit, too, as semantic processing at either the encoding *or* at the retrieval locus resulted in a recall detriment.) That youngsters could process semantic cues in their nonimpaired modality led us to postulate a theoretical model that received more attention in the regular cognitive literature than it did in the LD literature. We suggested that a single cognitive system subserved all forms of processing but that there exist modality-specific pathways to access it. We reasoned that a specific memory impairment was to be understood within the context of damage to one of the modality-specific pathways leading to this single processing system.

Let us say something more about this single system theory because it will help those who are interested in understanding why we have come to our current perspective. The singular cognitive system theory was congruent with our findings, but it was not the only theory that could accommodate them. We considered the possibility that separate cognitive systems coexist at any given point in development, but are not equally elaborated or amenable to cue utilization. According to this view, cognitive processes were seen as modular computational devices, operating only on some parts of the system at a given point in development. For example, inferential reasoning may appear in some domains of knowledge much earlier than in others and therefore operate only on knowledge in those domains. The same with spatial skills, analogical and metaphorical reasoning, and so on. We found this view of isolated cognitive subsystems somewhat dismaying and wrote in our 1980 paper of its "dyseconomic" status as a theoretical construct, as it implied a duplication of processes in each knowledge domain and seemed to fly in the face of a lot of good cognitive research that indicated a consistency of processing across all knowledge domains. At that time we assumed that persons who were able to solve basic arithmetic problems could do so regardless of whether the problem was framed in terms of how many newspapers Johnny sold or how many apples Mary purchased. *Mutatis mutandem,* we supposed that persons who were poor at recalling digits would be poor at recalling dance steps, too. So in 1980 we were not about to suggest domain-specific cognitive systems, each containing its own basic cognitive processes. So our modality-specific pathways to a single cognitive system position were really a compromise. We alluded to the principle of parsimony to justify this position, as if parsimony has anything to say about the truth of a matter. (Lest one think that we believe parsimony to be unimportant, our position is simply that it ought never be invoked automatically to settle a scientific debate, because theoretical goals need to be considered before accepting the superiority of parsimony over an account that contains greater *organized complexity*.)

Now, nearly 10 years after this initial work, and with the benefit of logical analyses by theorists like Fodor (1983), we have come to a more radical position, one that we resisted taking in our early work; namely, that *all* cognitive operations initially emerge in the course of normal development within a specific domain (e.g., personally experienced knowledge, quantitative knowledge, etc.) and only become *transdomainal* (i.e., operative across all areas of knowledge) with development. And for many of us these processes may *never* become transdomainal!

Ability-related differences, according to this view, could be the result of differences in the way knowledge is represented in a particular domain and/or of the efficiency of the cognitive processes that operate on such knowledge. As we will try to show, the representation of knowledge in a given domain sets important constraints on the efficiency of cognitive processes that must access it. If a child who exhibits a poor visual memory when the task is to recall digits does not exhibit poor memory when the task is to recall dance steps, then our position is that asymmetries in the way digit and bodily kinesthetic information is represented could explain the unevenness in performance more readily than could a deficit in an underlying cognitive process that supports recall such as a retrieval failure. We make no claim that the poor performances of *all* children with LD on cognitive tasks can be understood in terms of poorly elaborated knowledge representations in the pertinent domains, only that some, and perhaps even many, of them can. As will be seen, this view raises interesting and troubling questions about the very nature of the phenomenon under consideration, viz., learning disabilities.

Recently, Joe Torgesen (1986) and Keith Stanovich (1986) reopened this debate when both raised the question of the *specificity* of impairment, one of the presumed hallmarks of a learning disability. But for now, we shall return to this excursion of the last 10 years of work so that our current position can be better understood.

Having convinced ourselves that subgroups of children with LD could be identified who would behave in a systematically different manner on a cognitive task, our next goal was to discover whether the observed differences were of a *qualitative* or *quantitative* nature. In particular, the question we asked was whether the poor performance of children with LD was the result of a breakdown in some fundamental processing mechanism (qualitative), or conversely, whether it might be the result of a less efficient use of the same mechanisms that subserved the performance of their non-LD peers (quantitative). Over a 2-year period, we conducted three new experiments that addressed this qualitative versus quantitative distinction in LD/non-LD memory performance. In the first of these studies, we assessed whether the memory disparity between these groups was due to differences in their locus of processing; for example, perhaps children with LD differ from those without LD in their encoding, storage, and/or retrieval processing. We employed a mathematical technique that we developed to separate processing that occurs at the time of encoding from that which occurs at the time of storage or at the time of retrieval. If there were qualitative differences in processing that underpinned group differences in memory performance, then we might expect to see asymmetries in the locus of processing, with children with LD omitting processing at one or more of the stages utilized by those without LD. We did not find this, however. The loci of the processing of those with LD looked very similar to that of those without LD, except that it was at a lower rate at each locus. There was not a missing locus or anything else suggesting a qualitative difference interpretation. (Naturally, this distinction between qualitative and quantitative processing is somewhat arbitrary, and it could be argued that quantitative differences at one level are themselves due to qualitative differences at a prior level. And the reverse causal chain is no less plausible, with qualitative differences at one level being the result of quantitative differences at a prior level.) In two related studies, we examined qualitative versus quantitative differences in the processes that support attention and automaticity. The details of these researches are beyond the scope of this discussion; however, they are available elsewhere for those interested (Baker, Ceci, & Herrman, 1987; Ceci, 1984; Ceci & Tishman, 1985).

Suffice it to say that these early studies bolstered our confidence that we were dealing with groups of children who performed in a *quantitatively* inferior fashion to children without LD but who were *qualitatively* fairly similar to them in their style of processing. The children with LD went through the same cognitive steps as did those without LD, though more slowly or less efficiently. To provide one example of the evidence that prompted us to arrive at this conclusion, Ceci (1983) published the results of the following experiments, designed to assess ability-related differences in so-called *automatic* and *purposive* processing. This contrast was chosen because it maps directly on to the qualitative/quantitative distinction mentioned above. Basically, automatic processes are thought to be impervious to all but the most severe environmental variations, whereas purposive processes, as you might infer from the name, proceed in fits and starts, and, unlike the all-or-none nature of automatic processing, are a matter of degree and can be measured along a continuum. According to Hasher and Zacks (1979), Posner and Snyder (1976), Tulving, Schacter, and Stark (1982), and others, deficits in automatic processing are due to nervous system insults, whereas deficits in purposive processing can be due to a number of sources, including motivational ones (e.g., the failure to deploy strategies that the child possesses) and knowledge-based deficits that constrain the effectiveness of processing effort. Automatic processing is supposed to be at an unconscious level and does not compete with on-line information processing, nor does it require limited capacity attentional resources; finally, it is not amenable to practice, education, or acculturation effects (Hasher & Zacks, 1979). In contrast, effortful processing is quite sensitive to practice, education, and so forth, and requires the allotment of on-line attentional resources to be completed. An example of automatic processing that nicely illustrates its biological nature can be seen in the case of those individuals who suffer from dense amnesias. When they are told a joke for the first time, they laugh quite loudly; the following time they are told the same joke, they report not having heard it before, yet they do not laugh at it as loudly. This is interpreted as automatic processing because it is beneath the level of awareness and no conscious strategy to remember is involved—yet the joke has obviously been processed to some degree because it influences their behavior (Jacoby & Kelley, 1987). If children with LD behave in a qualitatively different fashion from their non-LD peers, then it should be evident on automatic processing tasks, even when their purposive processing on these tasks is normal.

To examine this issue, we conducted a study whereby children with LD and their non-LD peers were asked to listen to a word and then name a familiar object that was depicted in a slide. Children's response latency was assessed as a function of the relevance of the word they were presented to the object depicted in the slide. Hence the words could serve as primes to help children name the objects faster—provided they were relevant. In one condition, 80% of the words were related to the objects in the slides (e.g., *ANIMAL: horse*), and the remaining 20% of the words were semantically unrelated (e.g., *ANIMAL: book*). In the reciprocal condition, subjects were exposed to 80% of words that were unrelated to the objects in the slides, and only 20% of the words were related. Figure 8.2 shows something quite interesting: When children with LD are presented highly related words (80%), they don't derive nearly as large an advantage from them as do their non-LD peers. The suggestion of what is going on is straightforward: When children without LD hear a word, they begin to generate associations to it in a conscious (purposive) manner. If any of these associations happen to be the name of the object depicted in the slide that is presented shortly after the word, then it will lead to faster naming times. Children without LD demonstrate large advantages when these words are related to the objects 80% of the time. (Compare their naming speeds to that of the neutral condition in which the word is simply "ready.") But when only 20% of the prime words are related, it does not behoove the child to pay attention to them because they will lead to the generation of unrelated associations that will actually increase the naming time of the object in the slide. Interestingly, children with and without LD perform comparably in the 20% related condition. It is less advantageous to attend to the words in this condition because 80% of the time they will mislead one. Yet all children reaped approximately 30 msec advantage in this condition, and they did not suffer the other 80% of the time! This suggests that they automatically processed all of the words, and when they were related to the objects, naming speed increased, and when they were not, naming speed did not decrease vis-à-vis the neutral condition. Congruent with this interpretation is the absolute magnitude of the advantage: It is almost exactly the magnitude that the children with LD gained when 80% of the prime words were related to the objects. In other words, they appear to be locked into an auto-

MEDIAN REACTION TIMES (in msec)

"Benefits" = Neutral Minus Compatible
"Costs" = Incompatible Minus Neutral

Condition 80/20

Age	Neutral	Compatible	Incompatible	Cost	Benefit
4	1814	1770	1820	6	44*
7	1361	1301	1398	37*	60*
10	991	832	1082	91**	159***
L/LD 10	1009	973	1014	5	36*

Condition 20/80

Age	Neutral	Compatible	Incompatible	Cost	Benefit
4	1823	1788	1819	−4	35*
7	1344	1301	1358	14	43*
10	988	946	999	11	42*
L/LD 10	979	943	982	3	36*

*p < .05
**p < .01
***p < .001

Figure 8.2. Median reaction times associated with naming pictures that were preceded with congruent and incongruent auditory primes.

matic mode of processing whereas children without LD can shift from purposive to automatic processing when the conditions warrant it.

On the basis of these experiments, we began to become convinced that what separated children with LD from their higher functioning non-LD peers as well as from their lower functioning agemates who were called slow learners was the result of a *knowledge × process × context* interaction. As you know, lots of good research over the years has identified language-based deficits among children with LD, with language/learning disabled children constituting the largest subgroup of all children classified as LD. It is not clear to us at this point in time whether the problems of these children are fundamentally of a linguistic nature (e.g., a congenital limitation on phonemic awareness could set in motion a lengthy negative learning history in which less vocabulary is acquired by these youngsters; hence their receptive and expressive skills suffer), or whether this language problem is epiphenomenal, sort of like assuming the puffs of smoke are what is driving the locomotive rather than merely symptomatic of some underlying source. Many candidates exist to fill the role played by phonemic awareness, such as memory, attention, and even abstract rule learning, though this latter presents real difficulties for the specificity assumption, we will argue. At any rate, because of these underlying deficits, the knowledge bases of children with LD may be less developed than those of their non-LD peers (at least in those language-related domains we studied), and this lack of development could set limits on how effectively they encode, retrieve, abstract, and infer in these domains. Because the question of how or why their knowledge bases are less developed is one we cannot answer, it is important to refrain from assuming that it is due to impaired cognitive processes at all, as such an explanation would not account for an interesting phenomenon: In most of our studies, children with LD can often be seen to exhibit normal cognitive processes (memory, attention, etc.) in some domains but not in others. Their performances in these domains suggest that they possess cognitive processes that would have been useful in the other domains, provided there existed sufficient knowledge in them for these cognitive processes to operate.

The nature of the knowledge base limitations of children with LD is often quite subtle and can easily be overlooked. For example, in one study we asked children to solve verbal analogies of the usual format:

TALL:SHORT:: (a) front:back, (b) hot:cold, (c) dead:alive, (d) married:single

As can be seen, all of the possible answers appear at first glance to apply because they are all antonymic. But it was found that most non-LD 11- to 13-year-old children instinctively select answers like "b," while the children with LD did not differentiate among the three distractors. (The reasons, by the way, are well grounded in linguistic theory; only "b" captures the continuous nature of the *tall-short* distinction. One cannot place the adverb *very* before *front, dead,* or *married*— except in a metaphorical sense of being *very dead* or *very married*.) We used a number of these subtle linguistic contrasts to build analogies, and discovered that children with LD were less knowledgeable than their non-LD peers on many of them and, consequently, appeared to be deficient in analogical reasoning. We are currently attempting to replicate this effect by using multidimensional scaling to infer how elaborately children represent concepts. Armed with the representation of knowledge of children with LD in various domains, we will give these same children various problems to solve utilizing these same concepts. It is expected that LD children, despite their overall poor performance, will perform as well as non-LD children when the concepts are elaborately represented.

In another investigation we asked LD and non-LD 10-year-olds to attempt to predict where, on a computer screen, a geometric shape that initially appeared at the center would terminate. If a circle appeared at the center of the screen, it might begin to move toward one of the four compass points, either a short or long distance; thus there were eight possible destinations. In the simplest problem type, there were eight possible configurations of the geometric stimulus, given by its shape (square vs. circle) × color (black vs. white) × size (small vs. large). It was a completely additive algorithm that drove the event. For example, the attribute "black" might indicate that the shape would travel a long distance, while "white" indicated it would travel a short distance; "squares" might indicate a leftward movement, while "circles" might indicate a rightward movement; and "large" objects might indicate a downward movement, while "small" objects might indicate an upward movement. So, if a large, black circle appeared at the center of the screen, its destination was given by the addition of the main effects for *size, shape,* and *color*. (In later studies, we got fancy and programmed multiplicative functions to drive the event and the results were always the same, though the absolute levels of accuracy at predicting where the event would terminate was much lower with these more complex algorithms.)

In addition to asking these children to estimate where the shape would terminate, we asked their peers to play a video game we developed. The game required children to try to capture butterflies or bumblebees by positioning a graphic net on the screen at the point where they thought the bee or butterfly would terminate. The bees and butterflies might be small or large and they might be black or white.

As can be seen, this video game was what is termed a *problem isomorph,* differing from the geometric shape task only in its concreteness and its linkage to children's video game knowledge. You may wonder what sort of knowledge children could have possessed about this game. Well, no specific knowledge, of course, as we developed the game ourselves and they experienced it for the first time in our lab. But children who play video games build a repertoire of strategies and heuristics that can aid them on nearly all video games. If you doubt this statement, try watching those children on a Saturday afternoon at the game arcades at your local mall when they try a new game. They seem amazingly quick at grasping what is required because so much of what is required is also needed for games they have already mastered. The point of this speculation is that placing the algorithm within the context of a video game elicits children's video game knowledge. In related work on prospective remembering, Urie Bronfenbrenner and we have shown that children's familiarity with video games was linked to their use of certain strategies (Ceci, Bronfenbrenner, & Baker, 1988).

In Figure 8.3 you can see what happens when we compared the children who were asked to solve the task as a geometric shape prediction exercise with those asked to solve it as part of a butterfly/bee capture game. Children with LD in the disembedded geometric shape task do not do very well, even after 750 trials, vis-à-vis the children without LD. In contrast, in the video game format, they perform about on par with the non-LD children. The interaction is equally striking

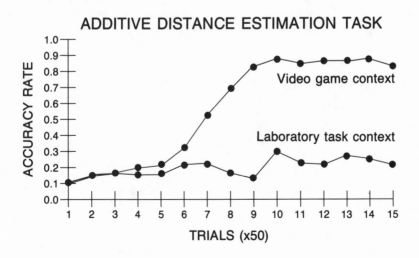

Figure 8.3. Children's mean proportion of accurate estimates of a moving object in game versus laboratory contexts (simple main effects algorithm).

for the more complex algorithms. The reason for the lower performance of the children with LD in the disembedded context is not clear and may be simply attentional. After all, these children were nearly adolescents, and their long and difficult learning history probably had already exacted its toll in the amount of attention they were prepared to devote to academic-type tasks.

In case you did not get one of the implications of these findings, let us spell it out: If we had assessed the multicausal reasoning of the children with LD only in the context of the geometric shape prediction task, we would have been led to a needlessly ungenerous estimation of their ability to solve multicausal problems in a probabalistic feedback environment. Clearly, they had some ability that was not evident on the geometric shape task, and the impression we have is that many other instances of superior performance among these children could be identified if we found ways to control for knowledge base differences between them and their non-LD agemates. Again, we see that there was not what one might regard as a qualitative difference between children with and without LD in the ability to use a cognitive process, in this case *multicausal reasoning*. Both groups were able to solve problems of identical complexity. What was obvious was that one group, namely the children with LD, were unable to solve these types of problems in a disembedded, some might even say *abstract* (though we hesitate to use that term because of its conceptual unclarity), format. It was a matter of quantity, not quality, in the ability to engage in this type of reasoning. Based on these sorts of findings, we regard the literature documenting deficits among children with LD in central cognitive processes such as reasoning to suggest not a true deficit in reasoning but rather a failure to use whatever reasoning capacity they have within knowledge-impoverished domains.

Lest we give the impression that all of our early studies conformed to this conclusion, we hasten to add that they did not. We also examined LD/non-LD differences on an attentional task to determine if the deficits of the children with LD were due to an automatic or a purposive processing deficit. Recall that according to this distinction, automatic processing is supposed to be at an unconscious level and does not compete with on-line information processing, nor does it require limited capacity attentional resources, whereas purposive processing requires the allotment of on-line attentional resources to be completed. We had expected that children with LD would be deficient at purposive processing but not at automatic processing, given our knowledge-based view of learning disablement. After all, it is purposive processing that is amenable to learning effects and education; automatic processing is assumed to be a by-product of neurological status and is thought to be relatively immune to experiential differences. If there is a neurological basis for learning disabilities, then how come they could perform well in some contexts but not in others? The results of earlier studies favored a more environmental explanation. As persuasive as this line of reasoning may strike one, we found just the opposite! Because the task that we designed was an interesting one, and because perhaps there are some features that we overlooked in our thinking, we will briefly describe it here. LD and non-LD 12-year-olds were first asked to play a video game that we programmed. It involved trying to steer a spacecraft to each of 20 planets, in a specified order. These planets were arranged around the periphery of a computer screen. If children could land the spacecraft on each of the 20 planets without being destroyed by missiles fired from alien craft, they would win the game. We designed it to resemble the sort of games kids play on their own. While kids played this game they were asked to wear a "pilot's headset." During the game they would hear words through this headset, but these words need not concern them now, they were told. Later, however, we would ask them to pay attention to these words and repeat them for us, but for now they were told they could ignore them and concentrate on the video game. Unbeknownst to the children, the game was rigged. No matter how adroitly they navigated their craft through the storm of alien missiles, it would be destroyed at a predesignated moment. And when this happened, there would be a colorful and noisy explosion on the screen. Kids loved it!

What the children were not told was that the words they were instructed to ignore bore a definite relationship to what was happening in the game. Each time a prespecified target word was announced in their headset, their craft would be destroyed by a missile. As we said, this was accompanied by a colorful and noisy display of their craft disintegrating. While the children played this game, we recorded their skin conductance levels to assess how aroused they were. As you might imagine, each time their craft exploded, their skin conductance level rose appreciably. Following three consecutive explosions, each triggered by the onset of this same target word in the headset, we administered a fourth trial during which the occurrence of the target word did not trigger an explosion. We wanted to find out if we had classically conditioned children's skin conductance to the onset of the target word. If their prior level of skin conductance when the target was paired with the loud explosion was recovered without the accompanying loud and colorful display, then we knew that we had associated the naturally evocative properties of the noise and color with the formerly neutral properties of the target word. This part of the experiment worked as planned, and we were able to demonstrate, for most children, considerable conditioning after just three pairings of the target word and the loud noise, so that when it occurred in the absence of the noise it still elicited a large skin conductance response.

Once conditioning was established for each child, we turned off the game and told them that they now should pay attention to the words being delivered in the headset. In particular, we asked them to repeat the words that were presented to one ear and ignore those being delivered to the other. At a 200-msec rate, it is exceedingly difficult to attend binaurally to words presented with an onset asynchrony of 20 msec; subjects are almost always able to focus on only one ear successfully. This was certainly true of these children, too. They could repeat the words delivered to their designated ear (counterbalanced right/left), and they were completely unaware of the words delivered to their nondesignated ear. We continued to record their skin conductance during this phase of the experiment. We were interested in whether children with LD would differ from their non-LD peers in their pattern of semantic activation. We determined this by measuring their level of skin conductance when a synonym or antonym of the target word was presented to their nonattended ear. We also assessed what happened when rhyme words to the target were presented to their nonattended ear. And we naturally compared these recordings to their level of response when these same words were presented to their attended ear (see Figure 8.4a).

Contrary to our prediction, children with LD did not appear to differ at purposive semantic processing—the kind measured by attending to synonyms presented to their designated ear. They performed equivalently to non-LD children in their level of skin conductance to all types of semantically relevant associates to the target word (synonyms, antonyms, etc.) as well as in their accuracy, number of interpenetration errors (reporting a word from the nondesignated ear as having been presented to the designated one), omissions, and latency. Interestingly, children with LD appeared to engage in much more purposive phonemic processing, as can be seen by their larger skin conductance responses to rhyme words presented to their designated ear. (In view of the fact that these children were diagnosed as "language-learning disabled," it should come as no surprise to find them poorer at auditory discrimination than the non-LD children, as indexed by their greater likelihood of processing words that were similar but not identical to the targets.)

It was in their automatic semantic processing (shadowing the nondesignated ear) that the two groups differed most seriously. This was a surprise to us, as we had debated Bob Sternberg about the normal course of semantic development—we argued that it was from automatic to purposive, and he had argued that it was exactly opposite, that automatic activation of a word's features could come about only after

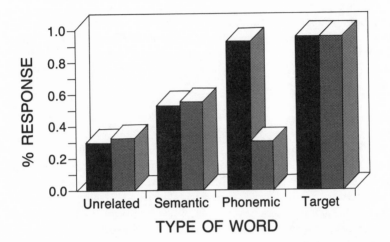

Figure 8.4a. Mean percentage of words associated with large SCRs presented to the attended ear. (Dark bars denote learning disabilities; hashed bars denote no learning disabilities.)

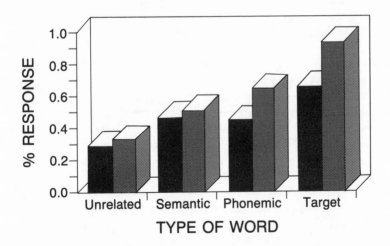

Figure 8.4b. Mean percentage of words associated with large SCRs presented to the nonattended ear. (Dark bars denote learning disabilities; hashed bars denote no learning disabilities.)

much purposive activation, much like other highly practiced behaviors in the course of being routinized. You can see from Figure 8.4b that children with LD did not engage in nearly as much semantic process- ing to the nonattended ear. Coupled with the above results, we con- clude that the children in this sample predominantly processed at the phonemic level, though they were not very adept at it. Perhaps their well-known difficulties in this area prompted them to overfocus on the sound structure of stimuli, to the near exclusion of semantics.

CONCLUSION

What is one to make of all of this? The answer depends, of course, on whether one hopes to synthesize these findings into an extant view of learning disablement with as much parsimony as possible or whether the goal is to use them as a springboard to challenge traditional con- ceptualizations of what it means to be a disabled learner. We propose the latter. With this goal in mind, let us suggest what the results may tell us about the nature of learning disabilities and about the kinds of children who have been participating in many of the experiments we carried out.

First, and foremost, it seems to us that these findings challenge the existing view of learning disabilities as an impairment in one or more basic psychological processes involved in understanding lan- guage, at least for some of the children. If a basic psychological process needed to understand language (e.g., phonemic awareness, memory, attention, rule learning) was truly impaired, then we might expect this impairment to be manifest across all language-based domains, not just some. One of the suggestions from the studies we reviewed earlier was that children with LD may be particularly impaired on language-related stimuli. If they are asked to attend, remember, or discriminate language- based stimuli, they perform poorly. Yet if they are asked to remember, attend, or discriminate nonlinguistic stimuli, they frequently perform on par with non-LD children. Our explanation for this asymmetry is that the manner in which linguistic stimuli are represented in long- term memory constrains how effectively one can attend, remember, or discriminate them. The more dimensions that cross-cut these stimuli and the more attributes and node structures that connect them and get cross-activated in their presence, the better they can be processed. Even something as basic as the speed with which a stimulus can be recognized has been shown to depend on how elaborately it is repre- sented in long-term memory. For example, people who know that *49* is a root number can recognize it faster (when it is tachistoscopically presented and masked at brief interstimulus intervals) than people who lack this knowledge, all other things being equal (see Ceci, in press, and Chi & Ceci, 1987, for other examples of knowledge-based constraints on the efficiency of cognitive processing).

If this knowledge × process × context account is extended to the case of children with LD, then they might be seen as having knowledge representations in some domains (especially language-related ones) that are suboptimal for certain types of processing. This would allow their success at using these same processes in other domains that appear deficient in language-related ones, and also account for how children presumed to have an impairment in some basic psychological mechanism could still perform adequately on many tasks that require this mechanism in nonlanguage exercises, such as the performance scales on IQ tests.

The second implication of the findings we have presented is that learning disablement may be seen as a state of functioning not qualitatively different from that of other children's. If we bear in mind that fairly substantial individual differences can be shown to exist on most cognitive performances, then the extent to which a language-based representation is elaborated might be expected to vary enormously across children at a given age. Suppose the degree of elaborateness of such representations is normally distributed. Then further suppose that the maximum efficiency of cognitive processes (itself distributed normally across children) is influenced by the degree of elaborateness of the knowledge representation they access. (We argue that the effectiveness of cognitive processes like memory and attention are directly tied to the way children represent the knowledge to be remembered or attended.) If correct, then we might expect large individual differences among children on cognitive performance, but this might be more of a quantitative difference in the degree of elaborateness of these representations and/or in the efficiency of cognitive processes that operate on them, rather than a qualitative difference in either. Notice that this argument is "promiscuous" in a sense because it is not tied to any particular level of processing such as the one just given—it works equally well if we talk about phonemic awareness being normally distributed across children, leading to differences in acquired knowledge.

If we are correct about this conclusion, then it raises interesting questions about the results of many researches, most notably those studies that have taken children that schools have identified as LD and demonstrated group differences between them and their non-LD agemates on so-called basic psychological processes. Such an approach ignores the possibility that the processing measures may not be measuring primarily the efficiency of the underlying cognitive processes per se, but rather a host of correlated knowledge-based and social-related factors. As Torgesen (1986) has pointed out:

> Thus, they [school-identified samples of children with LD] are not an appropriate sample on which to test theoretical models of learning disabilities. . . . We should recognize that statements about LD children based upon comparisons of school identified samples of LD children and other groups say more about the political-social realities of the placement process in schools than they do about the scientific validity of the concept of learning disability. (p. 405)

The *degree* of elaborateness may be correlated across various representations, yielding a large first principal component for generality of processing (with children tending either to possess impoverished representations across the board or enriched ones across the board). The mechanism that is responsible for this across-task generality may be due primarily to individual differences in children's linguistic environments, which in turn affect the elaborateness of their domain-specific representations, or to differences in the biologically determined limits of their memory, attention, or other cognitive processes. (The little behavioral genetic research that we are aware of suggests that the former explanation may not be the answer.) *Accordingly, there may be greater similarities among children with LD, so-called slow learners, and other children than has heretofore been assumed by LD researchers.*

And finally, we believe these findings bear on the question of the specificity of learning disabilities, at least for many of the children so labeled. If their difficulties stem from a qualitatively abrupt breakdown in a basic psychological process, independent of the level of elaborateness of the various knowledge representations upon which it operates, then there would be an expectation of pervasive performance decrements because such basic processes enter into a very wide array of performances. For instance, what task does not rely to some degree on encoding, memory, or attention for its successful completion? On the other hand, if the learning disabilities stem not from a breakdown in an underlying process, but from a limited knowledge base from which to construct a representation that can be accessed by basic cognitive processes, then we might expect to find children with LD who only appear to have a processing deficit and, given the right context or knowledge domain, are able to perform adequately.

Clearly, what we are proposing may be construed as a radical departure from existing views of learning disablement. However, by questioning such cardinal assumptions like specificity, as well as the qualitative nature of the disorder, we may be placing ourselves in a better position to understand disabled learning. In addition, by examining learning disabilities from an individual differences perspective that encompasses the interaction between knowledge representation and processing capabilities, we may be in a better position to face some of the theoretical and empirical challenges that await. And finally, by developing a concept of learning disabilities that is theoretically motivated, yet empirically based, we may emerge with a richer perspective that may, in turn, translate into more optimal educational advancements for disabled learners in years to come. Having made such allusions, it ought to be apparent how far we are from realizing them. Much remains to be learned.

REFERENCES

Adelman, H.S., & Taylor, L. (1986). Summary of the survey of fundamental concerns confronting the LD field. *Journal of Learning Disabilities, 19,* 391–393.

Baker, J.G., Ceci, S.J., & Herrman, D. (1987). Structure and process of semantic memory: Implications for the learning disabled child. In H.L. Swanson (Ed.), *Advances in learning and behavioral disabilities: An annual compilation of theory and research* (pp. 161–177). Greenwich, CT: JAI.

Ceci, S.J. (1983). Automatic and purposive semantic processing characteristics of normal and language/learning-disabled children. *Developmental Psychology, 19,* 427–439.

Ceci, S.J. (1984). A developmental study of memory and learning disabilities. *Journal of Experimental Child Psychology, 38,* 352–371.

Ceci, S.J. (in press). *On intelligence . . . More or less: A bio-ecological view of intellectual development.* Englewood Cliffs, NJ: Prentice-Hall.

Ceci, S.J., Bronfenbrenner, U., & Baker, J.G. (1988). Memory in context: The case of prospective remembering. In F. Weinert & M. Perlmutter (Eds.), *Universals and changes in memory development* (pp. 243–256). Hillsdale, NJ: Erlbaum.

Ceci, S.J., Lea, S.E., & Ringstrom, M. (1980). Coding characteristics of learning disabled and nondisabled 10-year-olds: Evidence for modality-specific pathways to the cognitive system. *Journal of Experimental Psychology: Human Learning & Memory, 6,* 785–797.

Ceci, S.J., & Tishman, J. (1985). Hyperactivity and incidental memory: Evidence for attentional diffusion. *Child Development, 55,* 2192–2203.

Chi, M.T.H., & Ceci, S.J. (1987). Content knowledge: Its representation and restructuring in memory development. *Advances in Child Behavior and Development, 20,* 91–142.

Fodor, J. (1983). *Modularity of mind.* Cambridge, MA: MIT Press.

Hasher, L., & Zacks, R.T. (1979). Automatic and effortful processing in memory. *Journal of Experimental Psychology: General, 108,* 356–388.

Jacoby, L.L., & Kelley, C. (1987). Unconscious influences of memory for a prior event. *Personality and Social Psychology Bulletin, 13,* 314–336.

Posner, M., & Snyder, C.R. (1976). Attention and cognitive control. In. P.M.A. Rabbitt (Ed.), *Attention and performance 4* (pp. 136–162). New York: Academic Press.

Stanovich, K.E. (1986). Cognitive processes and the reading problems of learning disabled children: Evaluating the assumption of specificity. In J. Torgesen & B.Y.L. Wong (Eds.), *Psychological and educational perspectives on learning disabilities* (pp. 87–131). New York: Academic Press.

Torgesen, J.K. (1986). Learning disabilities theory: Its current state and future prospects. *Journal of Learning Disabilities, 19,* 399–407.

Tulving, E.E., Schacter, D.L., & Stark, H.A. (1982). Printing effects in word-fragment completion and independent recognition memory. *Journal of Experimental Psychology: Learning, Cognition, and Memory, 8,* 336–342.

9. Assisted Assessment: A Taxonomy of Approaches and an Outline of Strengths and Weaknesses

JOSEPH C. CAMPIONE

In the recent critiques of the effectiveness of American schools, both instructional and assessment practices have come under strong attack. The crux of the matter is that there is a considerable amount of evidence that by the middle grade-school years, the majority of students have acquired many of the basic skills involved in reading (decoding), writing (producing a passable essay), and arithmetic (executing computational algorithms), but seem not to understand those activities in a way that allows them to progress beyond entering levels and become truly proficient. This predicament, common enough among regular division students, is even more pronounced among students in special education settings. The further argument is that this pattern is in good part a consequence of the way in which standard instruction is organized, and that it is then reinforced by accepted assessment practices.

Our recent research activities have centered on the development of novel approaches to instruction and assessment that can overcome

Preparation of this manuscript was supported by Grant No. P01HD-05951-17.

the limitations we see as characterizing much of current practice. The goal is to develop an overall theoretical framework within which the two sets of activities can be integrated. In this chapter, we concentrate primarily on the work we and others have done in the assessment realm, with some discussion of the implications of that work for instructional practice.

Since the inception of the testing movement at the turn of the century, the goals of assessment have remained the same. The idea is to develop tests that will generate descriptions of individual learners in terms of their strengths and weaknesses that will (a) predict how well they are likely to do in academic settings and (b) inform the development of instructional programs that can facilitate the performance of those predicted to experience particular difficulties.

Assessment practices have come under attack for both their predictive and prescriptive features. In the context of prediction, it has been argued that they are likely to misclassify students who come from nonmajority cultural backgrounds. Standard tests rest on the assumption that all students have had equivalent opportunities to acquire the information and skills probed for on those tests. To the extent that this assumption is not true, and it frequently is not, any inferences drawn from those tests are problematic. In the context of the relation between assessment and instruction, typical tests have been criticized in two, almost contradictory, ways. On one level, it is argued that typical ability and achievement tests *do not* inform instruction, that is, they do not provide the kinds of diagnoses needed to build instructional programs that can overcome student weaknesses. At the same time, there are concerns that those tests *do* influence instruction, albeit in a negative way. Students, teachers, schools, and so forth, are evaluated in terms of performance on standardized, norm-referenced tests. As we argue below, both the structure and content of those tests help shape and reinforce some of the negative aspects of traditional instruction.

In the area of special education, tests serve simultaneously to identify students to be assigned to remedial programs and to define the nature of the disability different children possess. Both legal and scientific definitions of various kinds of academic problems (mental retardation, distinct kinds of learning disabilities, etc.) are defined in reference to standard assessment instruments; performance on those tests serves as the basis for student labeling and influences the likelihood that the student will be assigned, for example, to a special education program. Beyond classification, the tests also function to suggest forms of treatment. For example, some students who are having difficulty learning to read may, on the basis of standard ability tests, be found wanting in their auditory sequencing skills. As a consequence, they may be given practice on items designed to sharpen those skills, with the hope that such training will result in improved reading ability. We have labeled this step, from diagnosis to intervention, the "leap to instruction" phenomenon, and have argued that the action is seldom easy to defend (Brown & Campione, 1986a, 1986b).

To improve upon the predictive and, particularly, prescriptive aspects of tests requires an understanding of the component skills and processes involved in the target academic tasks and the ways in which they contribute to successful or unsuccessful performance. It is only when we have a strong theory of the cognitive underpinnings of a given task, along with indications of likely sources of individual differences in their execution, that we can begin to build a diagnostic test. If, according to some theory, it is assumed that processes A, B, and C are involved in effective reading performance, and that skilled and unskilled readers differ most dramatically in use of B, the B should be a main target of assessment. These kinds of theoretical analyses serve to highlight *what* should be evaluated. Of course, theorists will differ in their analyses and hence spotlight different skills for measurement—the utility of the tests can then also serve as a way of evaluating the theories.

In addition to the what of testing, there is also the *how*. Even after we have decided to probe for process A, how do we assess it? In this chapter we will be concerned with two sets of issues. One has to do with the *degree of support* testees receive. Skills can be measured in situations where students work unaided on sets of items, and are given but a single chance to demonstrate their proficiency (static tests). The contrast here involves cases where students are given some form of help designed to maximize their performance, with this aided, maximal level taken as providing the clearer picture of student ability (dynamic tests). The second feature, the *degree of contextualization* of the assessment, involves two subthemes. To illustrate, assume that the ability to "identify main ideas" is deemed central to reading and writing. That skill can then be measured as either a relatively isolated activity, typically with specially prepared materials, or in the actual context of reading a text for meaning or producing an essay. A second issue concerns the degree of generality one assumes. If "finding the main idea" (or "auditory sequencing") is regarded as a fairly general characteristic, any measurement in any context will be acceptable. If, however, the ability to identify main ideas is regarded as varying within individuals over tasks (some may do it well while reading someone else's text but less well when producing or evaluating their own), the specific match between the target and testing settings takes on much more significance.

The majority of extant tests involve static assessment. Intelligence and ability tests also assume considerable generality of the processes under evaluation. And it is easy to see why this is the case; these are the most pleasant assumptions a test developer can make. Static tests, as opposed to dynamic ones, are much less complex to generate. No aid is provided, social interaction between the tester and testee is minimized (though not eliminated—Mehan, 1973), objective and reliable scoring systems can more readily be implemented, and norming is much simpler. The assumption of generality also makes life easier, as the specific context does not become a major concern. Evaluating a given process in one context provides information about its operation in all, or many, others. As a result, a small number of tests can be used to generate a considerable amount of information.

Assessment is of course not the whole story. Even if satisfactory and theoretically defensible assessment instruments have been designed, there remains the problem of translating test results into suggestions for remediation. A good assessment may well highlight the strengths and weaknesses an individual or group of individuals possesses, and hence may indicate the *contents* of an appropriate instructional program, but it cannot do that in the absence of a theory of learning and instruction that can be used to guide the way in which both the assessment and instructional enterprises are implemented. As we have indicated elsewhere (Brown et al., 1986a), prevailing views about the nature of individual differences in academic aptitude and about the nature of human learning have had profound effects on the identification and treatment of children with learning problems, be they called mentally retarded or learning disabled.

In the next sections, we outline what we see as some of the weaknesses of standard instruction and assessment. We also point to some recent attempts to generate alternatives designed to overcome those problems. In this context, we highlight the role of *supportive social contexts* for learning and their place in both instruction and assessment.

Our main goal in this paper is to summarize and organize a family of new approaches to assessment, generically referred to as *dynamic assessment,* that have been developed as alternatives to standard assessment practices. We want to explore the ways in which the various approaches to dynamic assessment can influence classification of students, perception of student abilities, and instructional practices. The defining feature of these approaches is a reliance on process, rather than product, information. In our treatment, we will be concerned with two aspects of dynamic assessment: (a) whether the skills assessed are assumed to be *domain general* or *domain specific* and (b) whether the assessment is structured in a formal, *standardized* fashion or in a more opportunistic, *clinical* way. Before turning to the assessment issue, we review some concerns with instructional practices.

TRADITIONAL INSTRUCTIONAL PROGRAMS: CRITICISMS

Elsewhere (Brown & Campione, in press; Campione, Brown, & Connell, in press), we have summarized some of the limitations of standard instructional practices that contribute to findings that students come to be able to perform sets of basic skills on demand, but do not acquire a firm conceptual grasp of the goal of those activities. They can perform the necessary subskills or algorithms on demand, for example, when cued on a standard test, but without understanding their significance, they are not in a position to use the skills flexibly. It is our hypothesis that this result is explainable in terms of a number of features of typical instructional practices.

Throughout the curriculum, there is an emphasis on *direct instruction* with strong *teacher control*—the teacher lectures and the students listen. There is little discussion and few opportunities for students to contribute their own feelings, ideas, or concerns during the course of instruction. This tendency, present in reading and social studies courses, is most pronounced in mathematics, where teachers routinely work out problems on the board and then have the students work independently on related examples (Stodolsky, 1988).

With the students forced into a passive role, and not encouraged to contribute their own comments, there is little occasion for the teacher to engage in the kind of *on-line diagnosis* of individual student capabilities. Teachers respond by proceeding through their lesson sequences following what Putnam (1987) calls a curriculum script; it is the preset curriculum that guides selection of instructional goals and content, not student progress.

There is a strong tendency for lower level skills to be taught before higher level understanding, as if they were separable, leading children to misunderstand the goal; they come to believe that reading *is* decoding, that math consists *only* of running off well-practiced algorithms, and so forth. There seem to be two general assumptions underlying this sequence. One is that unless basic level skills are mastered, students cannot acquire higher level ones. An alternative is that higher level skills will emerge automatically from mastery of the basic skills.

Another consistent feature of much instruction is an emphasis on subskills. Many academic tasks, such as reading for meaning, are complex; and for purposes of instruction it is deemed necessary to make them more manageable for novice learners. Frequently, this means analyzing the global task into the discrete subskills that are assumed to be the components of the overall task. Instruction then focuses on those subskills, and students practice them in relative isolation from the real goal of the activity, such as reading for meaning.

This emphasis on subskills also results in a lack of explicit instruction regarding the more complex and global strategies that expert studiers deploy flexibly. As one example, analyses of the comprehension process have identified an impressive array of such tactics, ones that are acquired by extremely capable students in the absence of explicit instruction. These activities, such as summarizing and paraphrasing what one has just read, anticipating the author's argument, and so forth, allow students both to extend their comprehension and to monitor its progress. (If one cannot summarize or if anticipations are disproved, this is evidence that comprehension is not occurring.) However, there is by now considerable evidence that less capable students do not acquire a variety of such cognitive strategies unless they are given detailed and explicit instruction in their use (e.g., Campione, Brown, & Ferrara, 1982; Rohwer, 1973). It is also true that the more complex the strategy in question, the more explicit the instruction needed, even for more capable students (Brown, Bransford, Ferrara, & Campione, 1983; Day, 1986). The idea that complex problem-solving strategies will emerge from instruction aimed at instilling their constituent subskills is difficult to defend. Worse, even when practice in understanding is finally provided, frequently it too is treated as consisting of decomposed skills (summarizing, inferring, etc.). Such activities are presented as ends in themselves, rather than as a means to a more meaningful end. Little attention is paid to the flexible or opportunistic use of strategies in appropriate contexts.

Unfortunately, this emphasis on skill training is particularly stressed for low achieving students, for whom explicit instruction in understanding is particularly necessary. Higher level strategies are rarely taught. Students perceived by their teachers as less capable are seldom asked to engage in sophisticated reasoning processes, but instead are required in the case of reading to concentrate on pronunciation rather than understanding a text (e.g., Collins, 1980), or doing simple computations rather than deploying new procedures (e.g., Petitto, 1985). Hence, weaker students seldom get to practice the higher level skills they are most unlikely to acquire spontaneously.

TRADITIONAL INSTRUCTIONAL PROGRAMS: CONSEQUENCES

Given this educational history, it is not surprising that students have difficulty understanding and orchestrating their own learning.

Many students acquire a distorted view of what academic tasks are and hence come to believe that reading is decoding, that math is executing algorithms, that writing is neatness, and so forth. They come to view the syntax of the domain, rather than its semantics, as its core concept (Resnick, 1982). Given that many of the practices underlying these views are particularly emphasized for students having academic problems, it is not surprising that these students are most likely to have distorted views of the main goals of schooling. They suffer from problems in two main arenas. Their *knowledge* of the domains is faulty, and they experience particular difficulties attempting to *monitor* and *regulate* their on-line learning and problem-solving attempts. In contemporary parlance, they have problems with metacognition (Brown et al., 1983).

On the positive side, there is growing consensus that interactive learning environments, in which the goal is to enhance students' conceptual understanding of the semantics, or the meaning, of procedures, produce more insightful *intentional learners*. One example of such an approach is reciprocal teaching of reading comprehension (Brown & Palincsar, 1982, in press; Palincsar & Brown, 1984), and other examples have been reviewed by Collins, Brown, and Newman (in press). Although we will not go into detail here, reciprocal teaching involves a guided cooperative learning environment in which students take an active part in discussions designed to improve their reading comprehension. As we indicate below, that involvement affords teachers the opportunity to do on-line evaluation of individual student competence and to provide tailored instruction designed to enhance that competence.

TRADITIONAL ASSESSMENT PRACTICES: CRITICISMS

Students are subjected to a variety of tests during their school careers. As a general cut, we might distinguish between ability or intelligence tests on the one hand and content area (reading, mathematics, social studies, etc.) tests on the other. These tests are designed to play different roles and to provide different kinds of information. Individual students, particularly those who are candidates for special education programs, are most directly affected by intelligence and ability tests, but all students are affected, at least indirectly, by content area evaluations. The tests also lead to different kinds of problems and different types of criticisms. For example, intelligence tests are criticized because they may give a distorted view of *individual learners,* area tests because they lead to a slanted view of *academic domains.* In some cases, the tests are criticized from opposite ends of some continuum. Intelligence tests are criticized because they do not influence instruction, content area tests because they are overly influential. Intelligence tests are challenged because they may underestimate the potential of some students, area tests because they may paint too optimistic a picture of student progress. Although the criticisms differ, it is our view that the underlying causes are the same in both cases. These include a reliance on static, product-based tests, inappropriate levels of description, and the decontextualized nature of the evaluations. In the next sections, we consider these factors and their impact on the different tests.

Ability and Intelligence Tests

Ability and intelligence tests have been criticized in terms of both their predictive and prescriptive properties. Their larger success is in terms of identifying students likely to have particular problems dealing with school learning. Correlations between intelligence test scores and scholastic achievement are consistently high, not surprising as they were developed with that criterion in mind. However, even in the case of prediction, their success is limited, notably when children of poverty are involved. In the case of providing profiles of abilities that can be used to design interventions tailored to the needs of particular students or groups of students, they have been considerably less successful. And finally, they provide a pessimistic view of students who perform poorly. Elsewhere (Campione & Brown, 1987) we have reviewed some hypotheses that might account for the limitations.

Static, Product-Based Evaluation.   Standard ability tests are geared to establishing students' current levels of performance but yield no direct evidence abut the processes that underlie that competence. They may tell us where someone is at a given point in time, but not how that person got there. In this sense, they provide at best a partial picture of student capabilities, a point made nicely by Vygotsky (1978), who, in his discussion of the zone of proximal development, noted that static tests do not provide information about

> those functions that have not yet matured but are in the process of maturation, functions that will mature tomorrow but are in the embryonic stage. These functions could be called the "buds" or "flowers" rather than the fruits of development. The actual developmental level characterizes mental development retrospectively, while the zone of proximal development characterizes mental development prospectively. (pp. 86–87)

Vygotsky's notion is of a testing environment, incorporating some kind of social support, that will create a zone of proximal development in which students will be able to demonstrate the embryonic skills not tapped by static test procedures. In his view, it is the observation of these nascent skills that provides better estimates of an individual's potential for proceeding beyond current competence. Without such information, the likelihood of misclassifying students in increased. Particularly liable to be misclassified are students who have not had the opportunity to acquire the skills and knowledge assessed on standard tests (Campione et al., 1982; Feuerstein, 1979; Vygotsky, 1978). In addition, without any way of articulating the processes that may have operated, or failed to operate, to produce a given level of performance, it is not possible to determine how to devise an intervention to improve that performance.

Level of Description and Degree of Contextualization.   Although standard ability tests are product based, it is nonetheless the case that they are frequently interpreted in terms of sets of psychological processes. It is these inferred processes that are sometimes the basis for intervention attempts (Brown & Campione, 1986a). The problem is that the identified processes tend to be vague abstractions, drawn from a particular psychological theory, which are not readily relatable to performance on school tasks such as reading or mathematical problem solving. Hence, there are no specific suggestions for dealing with the student who is having trouble reading and/or doing mathematics.

This is not to say that nothing is done; the question is whether it is appropriate. The processes that emerge from standard ability tests are typically assumed to be quite general ones that operate in many, if not all, academic domains. The belief is in the centrality of general, decontextualized reasoning skills. This invites the conclusion that instruction aimed directly at those processes will have widespread effects throughout the curriculum—the leap to instruction (Brown & Campione, 1986a). If the analysis were correct, of course, enhancing those skills *would* represent an efficient way to remedy simultaneously a number of academic difficulties. However, this also leads to an approach that can displace alternatives aimed at teaching more domain-specific skills and competencies—students in resource rooms may practice their auditory sequencing skills, *rather than* skills associated with, say, reading comprehension.

Static Nature of Evaluation.   Another concern with ability tests stems from the conclusions that tend to be drawn. The result of assessment is frequently taken as providing a relatively permanent characterization of the individual in question. The classifications that result, already presumed to reflect general intellectual ability, are further regarded as fixed and unlikely to change. These expectations free teachers and schools from some of the responsibility for effective remediation; they also have a long history:

> I have always believed that intelligence can, to some extent, be taught, can be improved in every child, and I deplore the pessimism that this question often evokes. There is a frequent prejudice against the educability of intelligence. The familiar proverb which says, "When we are stupid, it is for a long time," seems to be taken for granted by unscrupulous teachers. They are indifferent to children lacking intelligence; they don't have any sympathy for them, or even respect, for their intemperance of language is such that they would say "this is a child who will never do anything . . . he is not gifted, not intelligent at all." I have too often heard this uncautious language.
>
> I remember that during my Baccalaureate exam, one examiner, horrified by one of my answers, declared that I will never have the mind for philosophy. Never! What a big word! Some contemporary philosophers seem to have given their moral support to such lamentable verdicts, asserting that intelligence is a fixed quantity, a quantity which cannot be increased. We must protest and react against this brutal pessimism and show that it has no foundation.
>
> If it were not possible to change intelligence, why measure it in the first place? "Après le mal, le remède." Diagnosis is crucial but remedy must follow. (Binet, 1909, from Brown, 1985, translation)

Despite Binet's impassioned plea, the view of intelligence as fixed and immutable continues to be held by many.

Content Area Tests

Content area tests differ from ability tests most obviously in the specificity of their content; they are geared toward particular academic domains. While the specific criticisms differ, their source remains the same.

Static, Product-Based Evaluation.   As with ability tests, a major criticism of content area tests includes the point that by resting on a purely product-based assessment approach, they are silent on the processes involved in the acquisition of those products. There are several paths to getting a correct answer on a test, and unless those can be distinguished, the assessment has the potential for providing misleading information. In contrast to the situation with ability tests, where the concern is that some students may get an item *wrong* for the wrong reason, thereby *underestimating* the competence of an individual, with content tests, the greater concern is that some get the item *right* for the wrong reason. There is by now good reason to believe that typical content area tests can provide a distorted view of progress by *overestimating* the capabilities of many students. Further, by so doing they reinforce some of the negative features of traditional educational practice that we reviewed earlier.

Interestingly, a major mechanism for these effects is the argument that, in contrast to having no effect on instruction, content area testing drives instruction. Students, teachers, and school districts are evaluated against performance on standardized tests, and considerable time is spent preparing students to take those tests. The items tested are in good part those that are taught, and what is taught helps to define, for students and teachers, the nature of the domain in question.

Level of Description and Degree of Contextualization.   If ability tests emphasize general, global processes, area tests go to the other extreme. They focus on the many subskills assumed to be involved in effective performance within the domain. The questions are whether (a) the skills as tested are in fact relevant to the actual domain and (b) if they are, whether students who can execute those skills as tested can actually use them in the service of the larger tasks of which they are a component.

Consider first reading assessment. In line with the notion that basic skills should precede higher level skills, as outlined above, tests at the earlier grades are heavily oriented toward phonics, as compared with comprehension, items. It is not until around fourth grade that this bias begins to change, and it is around this time that weaker students' performance begins to look particularly poor. Students with comprehension problems can do reasonably well on reading tests until this time, and it is not until around the fourth-grade level that their performance begins to diverge rapidly from that of more capable readers. If students do poorly on phonics tests in the early grades, they are given additional practice aimed at phonics skills, with an attendant further reduction in instruction having to do with comprehension.

Even at the upper grade levels, test structures continue to reinforce the subskills emphasis. The items designed to evaluate comprehension tend to tap skills in settings divorced from actually reading and understanding large segments of text. That is, the activities are tested as ends in themselves, rather than as means to the end of understanding what is being read. If reading comprehension is assumed to involve acts of finding the main idea, sequencing thoughts and actions, relating causes and consequences, summarizing, and so forth, then those skills appear on standardized tests. However, they appear as isolated activities, often in forms that are not recognizably related to normal reading. A brief, say three-sentence, paragraph is given, and the students' task is to identify the topic sentence—or they are asked to select an appropriate title from a set of nominees. It is not that these abilities are themselves unimportant; the objection is that the description of reading ability that results is in terms of performance on a large number of discrete subskills. Even if (some of the) activities are involved in effective reading comprehension, what is important is the reader's ability to combine and deploy them opportunistically as needed in response to different goals of reading, different text structures, and so forth. And these executive, megacognitive skills are not evaluated.

Testing is divorced from the context of reading large segments of text for meaning. Students are asked to perform on items similar to those that appear on worksheets associated with basal reader series; and it is quite possible to master those exercises without actually being able to read with understanding. Stated in another fashion, students are tested on their ability to perform the requisite activities, but are not tested on their understanding of those activities, for example, in terms of when or why they would be appropriate adjuncts to learning. Finally, students perceived to be doing poorly, in part by virtue of their performance on standardized tests, receive more drill and practice on the subskills appearing on those tests. And instruction aimed at more global comprehension skills is further delayed and reduced.

Similarly, mathematics evaluations are based on static tests assessing students' ability to run off algorithms, to solve problems displayed in a recognizable format, and so forth. Evaluations do not tap the extent of students' understanding of the procedures they are asked to execute. There is a tendency to assume that children who get the right answers know what they are doing, and those who fail do not. In addition, it is assumed that what a child does *now* on a test is a reasonable reflection of his or her knowledge, and that knowledge *predicts* or is equivalent to readiness to learn. It is those assumptions with which proponents of dynamic assessment quarrel. Students can be taught to run off algorithms in a purely rote or mechanical fashion, or they can be led to understand the rationale underlying those algorithms and hence something about the mathematical principles exemplified in them. The tests that are used to evaluate students clearly do not distinguish different possible paths to a correct answer.

The major problem with standard static tests featuring problems presented in canonical form is that getting the right answer does not necessarily indicate that a child knows what he or she is doing (Erlwanger, 1973). For example, Peck, Jenks, and Connell (in press) interviewed fourth through sixth graders who had just taken a standardized math test used by their school district for placement in appropriate instructional groups. On the basis of the interviews, they found four types of students—two of the categories are those that tests are meant to separate: (1) those who got the answers right and knew why and (2) those who produced incorrect answers and did not know why. But there were large numbers of students who fell into the other two classifications: (3) those who were right but who did not understand what they were doing and (4) those who were wrong but who did show evidence of understanding. On the basis of these interviews, Peck et al. reported that 41% of the students were inappropriately placed.

Of the latter two groups, Group 3 is the more interesting. Group 4 consisted of children who are scored wrong primarily because they did not conform to the strict rules of the game (½ is correct, ³⁄₆ is incorrect). Of more interest are students who appeared to have worked out the problem correctly, for example,

$$3 \tfrac{1}{3} - 2 \tfrac{5}{6} = {}^{10}\!/_3 - {}^{17}\!/_6 = {}^{20}\!/_6 - {}^{17}\!/_6 = {}^{3}\!/_6 = \tfrac{1}{2}$$

This child is in control of the algorithm. However, what happens if he is asked to discuss the answer a little, for example, by being asked if ½ or ³⁄₆ is larger? This student insisted that ½ is larger because "the denominator of ½ is smaller, so the pieces are larger and one of the great big pieces (½) is more than 3 of the tiny (sixth) pieces."

Having been suitably confused, the student had difficulty reworking the problem. This student, like a significant number of his peers, recognizes the problem type when presented in canonical form and can run off the algorithm correctly. However, he cannot resist counter-suggestions because he does not have a firm grip on the meaning of what he is doing.

Finally, as with reading, poor performance on mathematics tests frequently results in more practice aimed at perfecting algorithm use, again reducing the degree of attention aimed at understanding the underlying principles.

TRADITIONAL ASSESSMENT PRACTICES: CONSEQUENCES

By way of summary, we can point to several consequences of the structure and interpretation of ability and intelligence tests, on the one hand, and content area tests, on the other. Ability tests tend to be applied on a relatively limited basis. They affect directly individual students, or small groups of students, with their main role being to contribute to the classification and placement of students with special needs. In the case of content area tests, the situation is different in a number of ways. These tests are applied to all students and affect many, if not all, of them, at least indirectly. Because of mass testing, and the resultant use of, for example, matrix sampling procedures, little attention is (or can be) paid to the performance of individual students; attention is focused on the mean performance of groups of students (a school, a district, a state, etc.). The problems that result in each case, although different in many ways, result from the same general set of features.

Static, Product-Based Evaluation.   The emphasis on product, as opposed to process, information poses difficulties of interpretation in both cases. In the case of intelligence tests, if we assume that some testees may not have had the opportunity to acquire the knowledge and skills being assessed, there is considerable potential for underestimating those students' ability levels, leading to misclassification and mislabeling. In the case of content area tests, the failure to evaluate the reasoning underlying student responses can result in the opposite problem. Students can arrive at the correct answers for the wrong reasons, often having no real understanding of the operations they carry out.

In either case, the emphasis on product information results in the tendency on the part of some to assume that possessing the product information is equivalent to competence within the domain. Hence, teaching the specific information (knowledge) or skills (algorithms) contained in the tests is seen as the way to enhance competence— teaching digit span increases intelligence, providing historical facts makes one culturally literate (Hirsch, 1987), and so forth.

Level of Description and Degree of Contextualization.   We would argue that the levels of description associated with the two sets of tests are inappropriate, and again for opposing reasons. In the case of ability tests, there is an emphasis on quite general skills. Although there have been many debates about the existence of a general factor underlying intelligence, along with arguments about the needs for postulating specific factors, there is a general consensus that the number of factors is not very large. Those factors are then each seen to play a role in many aspects of intellectual performance. Individuals who perform poorly are seen as deficient in the operation of these general capabilities. The result of this view is that intelligence tests can provide a pessimistic, and frequently misleading, picture of labeled students, emphasizing that (a) their "disabilities" are in fairly general processing capabilities that can have widespread effects on a variety of academic tasks, and that (b) their potential for change is restricted.

The situation with content area tests contrasts sharply; there the items correspond to extremely specific and very narrowly defined subskills. By concentrating on subskills tested in canonical settings, content area tests contribute to a distorted view of the different academic domains (they reinforce the view that reading is decoding and that mathematics is the ability to execute familiar algorithms) and of the nature of delay within those domains (due to incomplete control of basic skills).

The structure of content area tests does influence instruction. Preparing groups of students to take and do well on such exams results in precisely the conditions we criticized about instruction in the earlier portion of this chapter. Subskills are practiced, the curriculum script (geared to the standardized tests) is followed, little on-line diagnosis of individual student progress is made, and so forth. Given this match between instruction and testing, it is likely that performance on those tests may overestimate the ability of many students. This elevated evaluation can then serve to indicate that the task of educating students is proceeding better than is actually the case.

Assisted Assessment: An Alternative Approach

It is in response to some of these concerns that we and a number of other investigators have turned to alternative methods of assessment. Dynamic assessment is the general term used to encompass a number of distinct approaches (see Lidz, 1987, for an overview), a term initially used by Feuerstein (1979). Others have used different descriptors, Budoff (1974, 1987a, 1987b) referring to learning potential assessment, Carlson (Carlson & Weidl, 1978, 1979) to testing the limits approaches, Bransford and his colleagues (Bransford, Delclos, Vye, Burns, & Hasselbring, 1987) to mediated assessment, Vygotsky (1978) to evaluation of the zone of proximal development, and we and our colleagues (e.g., Campione & Brown, in press) to assessment via assisted learning and transfer. The common feature is an emphasis on evaluating the psychological processes involved in learning and change. This is seen to contrast with standard methods of assessment that rely on product information. The argument is that individuals with comparable scores on static tests may have taken different paths to those scores, and that consideration of those differences can provide information of additional diagnostic value. The clearest example, of course, is of individuals who have not experienced a full range of the opportunities needed to acquire the skills or information being tested. And it is in this context—testing children from atypical backgrounds or children with school-related problems—that Budoff (1974), Feuerstein (1979),

and Vygotsky (1978) did their early work. It was also with these populations that our early work leading to a concern with assessment and
instruction was conducted (e.g., Brown, 1974, 1978; Campione & Brown,
1977, 1978; Campione et al., 1982).

The methods different workers have developed vary considerably
and reflect different goals. At one level, the concern may be with
increasing the predictive validity of the assessment procedure. Or it
may be with informing instruction. Although everyone aspires to both,
there are trade-offs that result in some procedures being more appropriate in one case than the other. Across approaches, however, the
common feature is an emphasis on individuals' *potential for change.*

In our own work, we have considered several goals of dynamic
assessment. The result is a set of approaches to dynamic assessment
that lend themselves to different sets of issues. We have been concerned
with attempts to improve both prediction and instruction. This schizo-
phrenic attack is not unique to us, but rather can be seen to characterize
the field in general. Before reviewing our programs of research, we
will outline a rough taxonomy of approaches to dynamic assessment
that have been proposed, and indicate some others that have not yet
appeared.

A Proposed Taxonomy

Three general dimensions have been considered. The first, which
we refer to as *focus,* looks at the competing ways in which potential
for change can be assessed. One is by observing the actual improvement that takes place following some intervention. An alternative is
to try to specify the processes that underlie any improvement and to
assess the operation of those processes directly. By *interaction,* we mean
the nature of the social interaction involving the examiner and subject.
That interaction can be conducted in either a standardized or clinical
fashion. And finally, by *target,* we indicate that dynamic assessment
attempts can be geared to either general or domain-specific skills.

Focus.   There are two general ways in which to evaluate potential for
change and hence determine whether that revealed potential has any
diagnostic value. The most common is via some form of test-train-test
procedure. Students take a particular test, are given some practice
and/or instruction on typical test items, and then a posttest. A number
of scores result from this sequence. First, there is the pretest score,
that which would normally be used for purposes of prediction or
classification. There are, in addition, data available from the instructional interaction itself. Next, there is the change score, or how much

improvement took place from the pre- to the posttest. Finally, there is the posttest score itself. Each of these is then a candidate predictor score, and the empirical question concerns which is the most useful. This is the general procedure used by, among others, Budoff (e.g., 1974), Vygotsky (see Brown & French, 1979), Campione and Brown (1984, 1987, in press), Carlson and his colleagues (e.g., Carlson & Weidl, 1978, 1979), and Embretson (1987). Below, we indicate some of the differences among these researchers.

The alternative approach to evaluating potential for change is to attempt to specify the processes involved in change in more detail and to evaluate their operation. That is, rather than looking at how much learning takes place in a given situation, we can try to specify the skills that underlie learning and evaluate them directly. The goal here is to end up with a description of individuals that reveals which skills are functioning smoothly and which are not being appropriately used. This profile can then be used as the basis for designing enrichment activities. In this approach, pre- and posttests are not necessary, although they could be incorporated.

Interaction.   For some, the goal is to devise a standardized protocol to govern the provision of help to students during the training portion of the intervention. That is, given a test-train-test sequence, the training experiences should be as standardized and consistent across students as possible given the restriction that it is impossible to completely standardize any social interaction. Others make the decision to resort to an unstructured, clinical interview approach in which the examiner is given considerable latitude in selection of both the tasks to be presented and the way in which he or she responds to the testee's statements and actions.

For those who choose to standardize the procedure (e.g., Budoff, 1987a, 1987b; Campione & Brown, 1987, in press; Carlson & Weidl, 1978, 1979; Embretson, 1987), the goal is to generate psychometrically defensible quantitative data that can be used for purposes of description and classification. Even here, however, there are differences. Budoff is concerned primarily with a gain score, the difference between the initial and final test performance (taking into account the pretest score). His argument is that gainer status will provide diagnostic information beyond that afforded by the pretest or other standardized scores, and he provides evidence in support of this contention (e.g., Budoff, 1987a). Carlson and his colleagues, as well as Embretson, focus more directly on the posttest score. Their belief is that the intervention provided between testing sessions will, for different sets of reasons, improve performance by minimizing the efforts of extraneous (motivational, misunderstanding of instruction, etc.) factors that artificially

reduce performance. The higher, less contaminated, levels of performance obtained on the final test should then provide more accurate
characterizations of subjects, and should result in greater predictive
validity; again, there is evidence to support this claim.

In our own work (Campione & Brown, 1984, 1987, in press), we
have taken still another approach. Our concern has been with measuring learning and transfer efficiency. Students are asked to learn new
rules or principles, and we provide titrated instruction, beginning with
weak, general hints and proceeding through much more detailed
instruction. We ask, not how much improvement takes place, but rather
how much help students need to reach a specified criterion with regard
to rule use, and then how much additional help they need to begin
to transfer those rules to novel situations. The idea is that these learning and transfer scores will provide more information about individuals
than competing static scores, for example, general intelligence or entering competence. Below, we review some of that work.

In designing the interaction between examiner and student, the
alternative method, championed by Feuerstein (1979) and the group
at Vanderbilt (e.g., Bransford et al., 1987; Burns, 1985; Vye, Burns,
Delclos, & Bransford, 1987), is to resort to a more clinical evaluation.
The argument is that the most sensitive assessments result when the
examiner, rather than being restricted by a standardized protocol, has
the flexibility to follow promising leads as they arise during the interview. A crucial feature of the interview is the ability of the examiner
to take advantage of cues provided by the student and use them as
an opportunity to probe in more detail an individual's strengths and
weaknesses. The goal here, rather than generating quantitatively useful
data, is to generate a rich clinical picture of an individual learner, one
that can be used to guide remediation attempts. It is also argued that
this is an efficient way to merge assessment and instruction. When the
examiner perceives a problem, he or she can select examples and
provide instruction designed to clarify misconceptions or show the
student how to improve his or her reasoning.

Target.   The goal of assessment can be evaluation of either relatively
general or domain-specific skills and processes. Some (e.g., Feuerstein,
1979) have concentrated on general skills (deficient cognitive functions, in Feuerstein's terminology), whereas others (e.g., Brown, Campione, Reeve, Ferrara, & Palincsar, in press; Ferrara, 1987) have been
concerned with assessments situated within a particular content area.
The competing assumptions are in terms of whether one wishes to
assess, and eventually modify, problems associated with intelligence,
or problems in more restricted cognitive skills (Brown & Campione,
1986b).

Examples and Evaluations

Although it is impossible to go into detail here, we would like to illustrate some of the contrasting approaches that have been taken, consider the goals encompassed in each, and review their strengths and weaknesses.

1. Standardized Interventions/General Skills

Efforts in this category are concerned primarily with devising methods to increase the predictive validity of the assessment process. The general approach is to work within the context of tests of fairly general abilities, and proceed on the assumption that assessments conducted at this level will provide information about individuals across a number of situations. The work of Budoff (1974, 1987a, 1987b) provides a good starting point. His approach involves a pre-post design with a standardized instructional component interspersed. His goal is to assess a general learning potential possessed by some educable retarded children that was not tapped by standard static tests. This potential is defined by the pre- to postgain score. Budoff originally distinguished *gainers,* those who show a marked pre- to posttest gain; *nongainers,* those who improve little; and *high scorers,* those who did well on the pretest. More recently, Budoff (1987b) has refined his scoring system to take pretest scores more fully into account, moving to a continuum of gain status rather than a tripartite distinction.

The main issue concerns the extent to which gainer status provides useful diagnostic and predictive information, and it does. For example, middle class children in special education classes tend to be nongainers, whereas lower class children have a high incidence of gainers. Learning potential status also predicts performance on a variety of laboratory concept-learning tasks and a specially constructed math curriculum. It also is related to successful adaptation to mainstreaming, the ability to find and hold jobs during adolescence, and a number of positive personality characteristics.

Carlson and his colleagues (e.g., Carlson & Weidl, 1978, 1979) and Embretson (1987) offer a related approach. Carlson and Weidl's method, referred to as *testing the limits* or the *integration of specific interventions within the testing procedure,* involves modifying the test context in a way designed to enhance performance. Again, they are concerned with standardized interventions designed to facilitate performance and provide a more sensitive index of a general intellectual capability. For example, groups of subjects may be given the Raven Progressive Matrices in the standard administration, or they may be required to verbalize the solution choice before seeing the alternatives or after making their choice, or they may simply be given feedback about the correctness of each choice. These modifications result in higher levels of performance on the Raven, increases that are seen to reflect modifications in subjects' understanding of the task, their greater comfort or reduced anxiety in the testing situation, and so forth.

The issue then concerns the predictive validity of the posttest scores, compared with the pretest scores. One expectation would be that the posttest results would be less useful, as the conditions under which the test norms were collected have been altered. However, Carlson and his colleagues report that the posttest scores are actually the more predictive. Interventions that facilitate the performance of individuals also lead to scores more clearly related to a number of criterion measures.

Embretson (1987) employs a standardized instructional component intervening between the pre- and posttest. She gave one group of subjects (a) a test of spatial ability, (b) training on folding three-dimensional shapes, and then (c) a readministration of the spatial ability test. Her subjects improved from the first to the second administration, and she found that posttest performance provided a better prediction of text editing performance than did pretest performance.

Some of our own work also fits into this category. We were concerned with a number of issues. The first was to test some hypotheses about the role of learning and transfer processes in students varying in scholastic performance. To do this, we had to devise measures of learning and transfer, and then investigate the concurrent and predictive validity of those scores. We worked with inductive reasoning tasks, such as letter series completion and Raven-type matrix problems. Subjects were given a series of static pretests, including tests of general ability (subscales from the Wechsler Intelligence Scale for Children–Revised [WISC-R] [Wechsler, 1974] and the Raven Coloured Progressive Matrices [Raven, 1956]) and a pretest on the test items. Following this they were given a series of learning and transfer sessions in which we assessed how much instruction they needed to learn in order to use a set of rules independently (learning score), and then how much instruction they needed before they could apply those rules in related but novel settings (transfer score).

The addition of transfer probes was dictated by a number of considerations. For one, we have argued elsewhere (e.g., Campione & Brown, 1978; Campione et al., 1982) that transfer performance is highly related to academic success. In addition, we also believe, with Moore and Newell (1974), that appropriate and flexible use of a rule or principle is the hallmark of *understanding* that rule; we also believe that the ability to understand a principle is related to future success. Both of these points dictate that transfer performance be included as a component of assessment.

Our first question was whether the learning and transfer scores would be related to general ability differences, and it turned out that they were (e.g., Campione, Brown, Ferrara, Jones, & Steinberg, 1985; Ferrara, Brown, & Campione, 1986). Lower ability, as compared with higher ability, children required more instruction to learn a set of rules to some criterion and needed more help to come to apply those rules to novel problems. Further, as the number of features distinguishing the learning and transfer problems increased, the performance decrements of the lower ability students became progressively more pronounced.

The second, and more crucial, issue concerned whether those scores would provide information beyond that obtainable from the static tests. To evaluate that issue, Bryant, Brown, and Campione (1983) took as a criterion measure the subjects' gains from the pretest to the posttest, and asked which scores or set of scores best predicted those gains. Across a number of studies, the results have been similar. If simple correlations are considered, the guided learning and transfer scores are the best individual predictors of gain; correlations involving static ability scores and gain average around .45, whereas the correlation between learning or transfer scores and gain are of the order of .60. And if static test scores are entered first into a hierarchical regression analysis, the dynamic scores added subsequently consistently account for significant additional variance (from 22% to 40%) in the gain scores. Also consistent across studies, the transfer scores always account for more variance than do the learning scores.

Critique.   The strengths and weaknesses of these procedures are clear. There is little doubt that they can lead to more accurate prediction and classification of individual subjects. All of the attempts, which feature interventions designed to facilitate performance, succeed both in improving performance and in showing that the heightened scores can possess more predictive validity than the unaided static test scores. That is true whether attention is focused on the gain from unaided to aided conditions (Budoff, 1974), posttest performance (Carlson & Weidl, 1978; Embretson, 1987), or on assessments of ease of learning and transfer (Campione et al., in press). The most important feature to emerge from our work is the particular sensitivity of transfer processes.

The major drawback to these approaches, in the context of assessment and instruction, is that they provide little information of direct use to teachers. We may be better able, through their use, to identify those likely to experience problems, but we cannot derive information to guide remediation attempts.

2. Clinical Interventions/General Skills

The goal of those in this camp, rather than improving prediction, is providing information about individuals that can inform instructional programs. The focus is more directly on sets of underlying cognitive processes that are presumed quite general, and the assessment is conducted in a clinical, opportunistic fashion that combines evaluation and instruction. In these applications, it is difficult to separate assessment and instruction. We would place Vygotsky (1978) and his treatment of the zone of proximal development in this category. However, the major figure here is clearly Feuerstein (1979). His Learning Potential Assessment Device (LPAD) has been developed in considerable detail, and the program is in wide use in the United States. Feuerstein's stated goal is to evaluate individuals' ability to profit from instruction, and toward this end the goal of the LPAD is to produce changes in fundamental cognitive processes and even to introduce new cognitive structures. He wishes to evaluate and remediate simultaneously.

To accomplish this, Feuerstein eschews the use of standardized approaches and argues for a flexible, individualized, and highly interactive format. He views the examiner as a teacher/observer and the examinee as a learner/performer. Crucial is the role of affect. A neutral unresponsive stance from the examiner is seen to reinforce the examinee's already negative self-feelings, and the provision of simple positive feedback is viewed as unlikely to be effective. Instead the examiner must function as a teacher, one who is responsive to the examinee in a multiplicity of ways—giving and requiring explanations, selecting examples (including repetition when necessary), summarizing progress, and so forth. The goal is not prediction of future behavior, but a statement of how modifiable the individual's structures are and where the individual's deficits lie. This is accomplished through the mechanism of a *cognitive map*, composed of seven parameters (content, modality, phase, operations, level of complexity, level of abstraction, and level of efficiency) that pinpoints the directions that instructions should take. The ultimate test of Feuerstein's approach rests in the improvements in academic performance that eventually result. Here the results are somewhat mixed, with some positive evidence being reported, along with some less successful attempts (see Bransford, Stein, Arbitman-Smith, & Vye, 1985, for a review and analysis).

Burns (1985), a member of the Vanderbilt group, has also employed this approach, using what she calls a mediated assessment procedure. This is in contrast to the graduated prompt procedure that we have used in some of our work (see previous section). A test-train-test paradigm is used. The defining feature of the mediated assessment approach is that the instruction that takes place is exactly that, intensive instruction in which the examiner does everything possible to teach the student how to solve the test problems. Emphasizing the relation between assessment and instruction, one criterion against which the mediated assessment procedure is evaluated is the examinees' performance both on the types of items practiced during the assessment session and on transfer items. Assessment and instruction are so strongly linked in this approach that unless the instruction has been effective in producing change, the assessment is seen to have failed.

Another aim of this approach is the development of individualized intervention programs based on the outcome of the assessment. Working with a stencil design task favored by Feuerstein, Vye et al. (1987) reported some success in this endeavor. Finally, one of the major criticisms of static tests, particularly those addressed at general intellectual functioning, is the view of the learner they generate. Low scorers are seen as having broad cognitive limitations and as unlikely to profit from standard instruction. Vye et al. (1987) also reported data indicating that teachers who observe dynamic testing sessions end up with a more optimistic view of the students than they do if they observe static testing.

Critique.   The goals of those who espouse this approach are more ambitious than in the previous case. And the criteria for their success, worthwhile improvements in academic performance, are more stringent. The main points to be considered in these programs are the same ones to which we have alluded throughout the chapter: (a) the level of description or generality of the target processes and (b) the degree of contextualization of the instructed activities.

Without going into detail, our main concerns are that the emphasis on very general skills, particularly in Feuerstein's case, leads to an enormous transfer problem. Assessment (and instruction) takes place with specially developed materials that intentionally bear little relation to school-like tasks, and it is quite possible for students to improve on their ability to deal with those tasks and yet show no appreciable gains in the academic disciplines. The instruction is divorced from the actual contents and contexts of schooling. As Bransford et al. (1985) pointed out, many of the gains achieved by those who have participated in the Instrumental Enrichment program (Feuerstein, 1980) have been on standardized ability tests. The evidence that gains in reading, writing, and arithmetic will follow remains uncomfortably slim.

In addition, there is the question of how we can evaluate the claim that the assessment process results in the identification of an individually tailored remediation program. Vye et al. (1987) provide evidence that, following mediated dynamic assessment, different children were seen to have different types of problems, and instruction based on that information resulted in clearly improved performance, that is, the assessment procedure did seem to be sensitive to individual differences and did lead to an effective teaching approach. The problem is that we have no way of knowing whether an alternative instructional avenue would have produced equal or better learning. That is, all that can be clearly claimed is that a responsive clinician, familiar with the domain in question and working one on one with a student, can help that student learn. The assessment cannot demonstrate the efficacy of a particular approach compared to alternatives.

Based on the reservations we have expressed thus far, the question is, what are the better alternatives? Our current bias is to situate assessment within particular academic domains. Whether the reliance is on a standardized approach to assessment or on a clinically based combination of assessment and instruction, it seems that we have come to know enough about basic academic subjects that we can design powerful techniques (Brown & Campione, 1986a) that can help overcome some of the limitations of traditional assessment and instruction. As examples, we offer two programs that have been developed in our laboratory.

3. Standardized Intervention/Domain-Specific Skills

In her PhD thesis, Ferrara (1987) extended our work on assessment via guided learning and transfer to the field of early mathematics. During the initial learning sessions, the student and tester worked collaboratively to solve problems that the student could not solve independently. The problems were simple, two-digit addition problems, for example, $3 + 2 = ?$, presented as word problems, such as:

> Cookie Monster starts out with three cookies in his cookie jar, and I'm putting 2 more in the jar. Now how many cookies are there in the cookie jar?

When the student encountered difficulties, the tester provided a sequence of hints or suggestions about how he should proceed, and Ferrara measured the amount of aid needed to achieve this degree of competence, that is, how much help does the student need to master the specific procedures?

Following this, Ferrara presented a variety of transfer problems in the same interactive, assisted format. These problems (see Ferrara, 1987, for details) required the student to apply the procedures learned originally to a variety of problems that differed in systematic ways from those worked on initially. Some were quite similar (near transfer: addition problems involving new combinations of familiar quantities and different toy and character contexts); others more dissimilar (far transfer: $4 + 2 + 3 = ?$); and some very different indeed (very far transfer: missing addend problems, $4 + ? = 6$). What was scored was the amount of help students needed to solve these transfer problems on their own. The aim of the transfer sessions was to evaluate *understanding of the learned procedures*. That is, the goal was both to program transfer and to use the flexible application of routines in novel contexts as the measure of understanding. Recall that one of our concerns about standard assessment procedures is their insensitivity to students' understanding of the routines they can apparently execute—many students get the right answer but for the wrong reasons. Inclusion of a transfer component in the assessment is designed to distinguish students who can use only what they were taught originally from those who, because they understand, can go beyond the specific problem types they have practiced and apply their routines flexibly.

After these learning and transfer sessions were completed, a posttest was given to determine how much the student had learned during the course of the assessment/instruction, the gain from pre- to posttest. The first finding was that the dynamic scores were better predictors of gain (mean correlation = $-.57$) than were the static knowledge and ability scores (mean correlation = $.38$). Further, in a hierarchical regression analysis, although the static scores when extracted first did account for 22.2% of the variance in gain scores, addition of the dynamic scores accounted for an additional 33.7% of the variance, with transfer performance doing the majority of the work; it accounted for 32% of the variance.

Critique.   The clearest conclusion that can be drawn is that this work reinforces the view that dynamic assessment procedures can be used to improve prediction. The learning, and in particular transfer, scores were more strongly associated with gain than were the competing static scores, and they also accounted for variance in gain even when the effects of the static scores were removed.

But we think there is more to say. There is also an important sense in which this effort combines assessment with instruction. In addition to helping predict how well individuals may do in some domain, it is highly desirable that the assessment process produce some payoff in terms of contributing directly to the instructional process. In one sense, the approach we have taken does this automatically—instruction is an integral part of assessment. While students are being evaluated, they are also being taught something about the domain in question. Further, the assessment involved not testing what students have already been taught, but skills that they have clearly not as yet mastered; they were asked to learn to solve problems that they could not solve at the outset. And they showed significant improvement in their ability to do just that. In the ideal case, the hints that are given are based on a detailed task analysis of the components of competence within the domain; as such, they provide a model of how one should proceed to solve the problems presented. If the hints are internalized to some degree, the subjects will have acquired relevant skills. That learning does take place is clear enough—in all the studies we have conducted, subjects have shown large gains from pretest to posttest.

Suggested Directions for Research.   From our perspective, an ideal way of integrating assessment and instruction would involve the interspersing of dynamic assessment sessions with regular instructional sessions. The assessment segments would provide current information on how quickly individuals were able to acquire and use new skills, as well as helping teach those skills. Although the sessions are time-consuming, the fact that the hints are preprogrammed makes it feasible to carry them out on a computer, and we have in fact done that successfully in our own work. As a result, the assessments could be done without taking up teacher time. The main point is that checking regularly for students' ability to use new resources would reduce the likelihood that they are acquiring progressive bits of knowledge that remain encapsulated and relatively inaccessible. If tests of current competence are solely in terms of the extent to which particular routines have been mastered and have become usable within familiar contexts, it is easily possible that some students will have acquired a repository of inert facts and procedures.

In addition to signaling that some students may be in particular difficulty, it is also desirable that the assessment process provide specific information about the kinds of help that individuals may need to advance more quickly. One approach is to develop sequences of prompts that can be organized qualitatively. In that way, in addition to determining the number of hints individuals require, information about the specific kinds of hints they need would also be available. This information could then be used to devise more specific remedial instruction. For example, Ferrara's hints included simple negative feedback (giving an opportunity for subjects to correct their initial response), verbal memory aids (reminders of the quantities involved in the problem), concrete memory aids, scaffolding (supportive prompts designed to help the child structure the problem), strategy suggestions, and so forth. Although we have not run enough subjects as yet to know if the additional information will be helpful, this approach is one we are currently pursuing. If such procedures could be devised, they would represent a way of combining the best features of the standardized (quantitative data) and clinical (qualitative descriptions) assessment procedures in a single package.

4. Clinical Assessment/Domain-Specific Skills

Our final example is the reciprocal teaching of reading and listening comprehension skills (e.g., Brown & Palincsar, in press; Palincsar & Brown, 1984). The reason for setting the approach within a specific domain is our feeling that it then becomes possible to select target skills to be taught and evaluated that are at an appropriate level of analysis—general enough to be applicable in many situations but powerful enough that they make clear contributions to learning. In the reciprocal teaching application, these guiding skills must also be concrete enough that they can be used to structure a discussion. Working within a domain also makes it considerably easier to contextualize the instruction in a reasonable way; the processes being honed are always practiced in the actual context of the academic task in which we are interested. The social nature of the procedure also makes it possible, as will become clear, to eliminate the need for reliance on subskills that characterizes many other approaches, again a way of increasing the degree of contextualization of the instruction.

Reciprocal teaching takes place in a cooperative learning group that features guided practice in applying simple concrete strategies to the task of text comprehension. A teacher and a group of students take turns leading a discussion concerning a segment of text they are jointly trying to understand. The dialogues are organized around four main comprehension-fostering and comprehension-monitoring activities: *questioning, summarizing, predicting,* and *clarifying.* These activities were chosen because they are known to facilitate comprehension and because they are used by skilled, but not unskilled, readers. The goal of the enterprise is to have the students become independent readers who use a variety of comprehension strategies opportunistically to aid their comprehension of texts. The task in each dialogue is joint construction of meaning. The strategies provide concrete heuristics for getting the discussion moving, teacher modeling provides examples of expert performance, and the reciprocal nature of the procedure guarantees student involvement.

The approach embodies five central principles:

1. When leading the discussion, the teacher actively models the target comprehension activities, making them explicit and overt.

2. The strategies are always modeled and practiced in the actual context of constructing meaning from text, never as isolated skills. They

are applied *as needed* to the task of understanding relatively extended segments of text. Although at the outset, individual students are not proficient at this overall activity, the social support provided by the teacher and the rest of the group makes the task a manageable one. It is this social feature of guided cooperative learning (Brown & Palincsar, in press) that makes it possible to practice nascent complex activities in an appropriate context, rather than as decontextualized isolated subskills.

3. Students are made aware of the nature of the strategies and when and how they are to be applied. There is little chance that they will fail to understand the significance of those activities given the explanations offered by teachers and the fact that the activities are used exclusively in the context of reading for meaning.

4. Central to our discussion here, the procedure forces each student to lead some of the discussions. In this role, students make their own level of competence apparent. Consequently, the teacher can engage in the kind of *on-line diagnosis* that is absent from traditional instruction, and provide instruction geared to the level of *that student at that time*.

5. Responsibility for the activities is transferred to the students as quickly as possible. As a student masters one level of involvement, the teacher increases his or her demands so that the student is gradually called upon to function at a more advanced level. Again, the emphasis on the teacher's need to monitor progress is clear.

Finally, as opposed to more formal assessment, the teacher's assessment of individual student responses need not be precise. The virtue of the procedure is that it is a regular component of classroom activity, taking place on a daily basis. As such, the teacher has many opportunities to monitor each student, and his or her judgments can reflect aggregations of a number of different inputs. The fact that there are many opportunities for evaluation means that no individual one is of particular significance.

This approach embodies some of the features of Feuerstein's program. Sets of processes involved in the task are specified; an environment is constructed in which students are observed as they engage in those activities; and the teacher acts as both an evaluator and a clinician, capable of discovering strengths and weaknesses and responding to student input by providing feedback, practice, and support as needed.

It is also different in fundamental ways. The processes that are targeted are chosen in reference to the academic domain in question, and the activities are always modeled and practiced in context. These two features conspire to minimize, or finesse, the transfer problem. As the activities are practiced in the context of reading for meaning, we need not be concerned whether they will transfer to that task. Also, if the program is successful, improvements are obtained directly on important school tasks rather than on processing skills that are assumed to be related to performance on those tasks.

There is abundant evidence that reciprocal teaching of reading and listening comprehension can be an effective means for dealing with poorly achieving students in the early to middle school years. The issue for future research is to establish that the principles that have been identified can be generalized to other content areas. This approach to integrating assessment and instruction rests on the ability to identify, in other areas, the kinds of activities similar to questioning, summarizing, and so forth, that are general enough to be widely useful but concrete and specific enough that they can both facilitate performance and support a discussion centering on the semantics of the domain. It is our belief that this is possible, and we have made beginnings in the area of elementary biology (see Brown et al., in press) and beginning algebra (Campione, Brown, & Connell, in press). It may not be the easiest thing to do (Brown & Campione, in press), but it seems worth the effort.

SUMMARY

Criticisms of educational practice have become increasingly frequent and strident. Many of the problems can be seen to be a consequence of the ways in which standard instruction and assessment are structured and of the interplay between them. In this chapter, we have reviewed some of the sources of the problems and argued that novel approaches to assessment—generically called dynamic assessment, which features the provision of assistance to the examinee—hold some promise for contributing to improvements in both assessment and instruction.

Dynamic assessment approaches emphasize potential for growth and can focus on either aspects of improvement that result from some intervention or on specified processes assumed responsible for learning. The skills assessed can be presumed either general and content independent or more specific and domain dependent. Finally, the assessment can be conducted either in a standardized fashion geared to the generation of quantitative data that can facilitate prediction and classification or in a more clinical mode aimed at providing a rich qualitative picture of individual learners that can be used to guide instruction.

Both the standardized and clinical procedures have their strengths and weaknesses. The standardized approaches provide quantitative data that serve a number of roles: (1) The dynamic scores are on occasion more predictive of other target behaviors than static scores obtained from the same test. (2) By focusing on potential for change and providing a forum most likely to reveal competence, they can help minimize the likelihood of misclassification of students, particularly those from poverty backgrounds. (3) The provision of assistance makes it possible to evaluate performance in settings just in advance of current capabilities, creating a zone of proximal development in which to gauge progress. In our own work, this enables us to look specifically at transfer performance, which we see to reflect *understanding* of newly acquired skills, a feature notably missing from static tests. (4) Teacher perception of student abilities is influenced. Teachers observing dynamic assessment sessions come away with increased confidence that the students can profit from suitable instruction. On the negative side, this approach provides relatively little information to guide instruction.

The clinical approaches hold more promise for contributing to educational practice, but are much more difficult to implement and evaluate. The data to support them are still lacking.

In either case, attention has been focused primarily on relatively general, content-independent processes. This may contribute to the weaknesses of each approach. Our suggestion is to concentrate on domain-specific, as opposed to domain-general, activities; and it is this tack we have taken in our more recent efforts. By situating research on assessment and instruction in the context of the major school areas, such as reading, science, and mathematics, it is possible to specify in more detail and with more confidence the skills and activities we wish to evaluate. Further, if we assess performance in the areas in which students are having difficulties and concentrate on skills known to be related to success in the domain, the problem of the leap to instruction is minimized. We thus avoid the problem of transfer. Finally, if we rely on assessments within domains, the view we provide of students may be a more optimistic one. The fact that someone does poorly in early reading does not mean he or she will have difficulty in mathematics or science. Given what we know of teacher bias effects, this is itself a worthwhile benefit.

Finally, the negative side to this view is that it requires that we develop separate assessment instruments and remedial instructional packages for each domain. Life would be easier if general skills were a major part of the answer. One test would do, one remedial curriculum would suffice for those having problems. Although we will follow with considerable interest those taking the general skills approach, it is our bet that progress can best be made by devising novel methods of assessment and instruction tailored to specific domains. We believe that dynamic assessment methods will come to play a progressively larger role in those activities.

REFERENCES

Binet, A. (1909). *Les idées modernes sur les infants.* Paris: Ernest Flammeron.

Bransford, J.C., Delclos, V.R., Vye, N.J., Burns, M.S., & Hasselbring, T.S. (1987). State of the art and future directions. In C.S. Lidz (Ed.), *Dynamic assessment: An interactional approach to evaluating learning potential* (pp. 479–496). New York: Guilford.

Bransford, J.D., Stein, B.S., Arbitman-Smith, R., & Vye, N.J. (1985). Improving thinking and learning skills: An analysis of three approaches. In J. Segal, S.F. Chipman, & R. Glaser (Eds.), *Thinking and learning skills: Relating instruction to research* (Vol. 1, pp. 133–208). Hillsdale, NJ: Erlbaum.

Brown, A.L. (1974). The role of strategic behavior in retardate memory. In N.R. Ellis (Ed.), *International review of research in mental retardation* (Vol. 7, pp. 55–111). New York: Academic Press.

Brown, A.L. (1978). Knowing when, where, and how to remember: A problem of metacognition. In R. Glaser (Ed.), *Advances in instructional psychology* (Vol. 1, pp. 77–165). Hillsdale, NJ: Erlbaum.

Brown, A.L. (1985). Mental ortheopedics, the training of cognitive skills: An interview with Alfred Binet. In S. Chipman, J. Segal, & R. Glaser (Eds.), *Thinking and learning skills* (Vol. 2, pp. 319–337). Hillsdale, NJ: Erlbaum.

Brown, A.L., Bransford, J.D., Ferrara, R.A., & Campione, J.C. (1983). Learning, remembering, and understanding. In J.H. Flavell & E.M. Markman (Eds.), *Handbook of child psychology* (Vol. 3, pp. 77–166). New York: Wiley.

Brown, A.L., & Campione, J.C. (1986a). Psychological theory and the study of learning disabilities. *American Psychologist, 41,* 1059–1068.

Brown, A.L., & Campione, J.C. (1986b). Academic intelligence and learning potential. In R.J. Sternberg & D.K. Dettermann (Eds.), *What is intelligence? Contemporary viewpoints on its nature and definition* (pp. 39–44). New York: Ablex.

Brown, A.L., & Campione, J.C. (in press). Interactive learning environments and the teaching of science and mathematics. In M.H. Gardner, J.G. Greeno, F. Reif, & A. Schoenfeld (Eds.), *Towards a scientific practice of science education.* Hillsdale, NJ: Erlbaum.

Brown, A.L., Campione, J.C., Reeve, R.A., Ferrara, R.A., & Palincsar, A.S. (in press). Interactive learning and individual understanding: The case of reading and mathematics. In L.T. Landsmann (Ed.), *Culture, schooling and psychological development.* Hillsdale, NJ: Erlbaum.

Brown, A.L., & French, L.A. (1979). The zone of potential development: Implications for intelligence testing in the year 2000. *Intelligence, 3,* 253–271.

Brown, A.L., & Palincsar, A.S. (1982). Inducing strategic learning from texts by means of informed, self-control training. *Topics in Learning & Learning Disabilities, 2*(1), 1–17.

Brown, A.L., & Palincsar, A.S. (in press). Guided cooperative learning and individual knowledge acquisition. In L.B. Resnick (Ed.), *Cognition and instruction: Issues and agendas*. Hillsdale, NJ: Erlbaum.

Bryant, N.R., Brown, A.L., & Campione, J.C. (1983, April). *Preschool children's learning and transfer of matrices problems: Potential for improvement*. Paper presented at the Society for Research in Child Development meetings, Detroit.

Budoff, M. (1974). *Learning potential and educability among the educable mentally retarded* (Final Report, Project No. 312312). Cambridge, MA: Research Institute for Educational Problems, Cambridge Mental Health Association.

Budoff, M. (1987a). The validity of learning potential assessment. In C.S. Lidz (Ed.), *Dynamic assessment: An interactional approach to evaluating learning potential* (pp. 52–81). New York: Guilford.

Budoff, M. (1987b). Measures for assessing learning potential. In C.S. Lidz (Ed.), *Dynamic assessment: An interactional approach to evaluating learning potential* (pp. 173–195). New York: Guilford.

Burns, M.S. (1985). *Comparison of "graduated prompt" and "mediational" dynamic assessment and static assessment with young children (Tech. Rep. No. 2). Alternative assessments of young handicapped children*. Nashville, TN: Vanderbilt University, John F. Kennedy Center for Research on Human Development.

Campione, J.C., & Brown, A.L. (1977). Memory and metamemory development in educable retarded children. In R.V. Kail, Jr., & J.W. Hagen (Eds.), *Perspectives on the development of memory and cognition* (pp. 367–406). Hillsdale, NJ: Erlbaum.

Campione, J.C., & Brown, A.L. (1978). Toward a theory of intelligence: Contributions from research with retarded children. *Intelligence, 2*, 279–304.

Campione, J.C., & Brown., A.L. (1984). Learning ability and transfer propensity as sources of individual differences in intelligence. In P.H. Brooks, R.D. Sperber, & C. McCauley (Eds.), *Learning and cognition in the mentally retarded* (pp. 265–294). Baltimore: University Park Press.

Campione, J.C., & Brown, A.L. (1987). Linking dynamic assessment with school achievement. In C.S. Lidz (Ed.), *Dynamic assessment: An interactional approach to evaluating learning potential* (pp. 82–115). New York: Guilford.

Campione, J.C., & Brown, A.L. (in press). Guided learning and transfer: Implications for assessment. In N. Fredericksen, R. Glaser, A. Lesgold, & M. Shafto (Eds.), *Diagnostic monitoring of skill and knowledge acquisition*. Hillsdale, NJ: Erlbaum.

Campione, J.C., Brown, A.L., & Connell, M.L. (in press). Metacognition: On the importance of understanding what you are doing. In R.I. Charles & E.A. Silver (Eds.), *Research agenda for mathematics education: Teaching and assessment of mathematical problem solving*. Hillsdale, NJ: Erlbaum.

Campione, J.C., Brown, A.L., & Ferrara, R.A. (1982). Mental retardation and intelligence. In R.J. Sternberg (Ed.), *Handbook of human intelligence* (pp. 392–490). New York: Cambridge University Press.

Campione, J.C., Brown, A.L., Ferrara, R.A., Jones, R.S., & Steinberg, E. (1985). Breakdowns in flexible use of information: Intelligence-related differences in transfer following equivalent learning performance. *Intelligence, 9*, 297–315.

Carlson, J.S., & Weidl, K.H. (1978). Use of testing-the-limits procedures in the assessment of intellectual capabilities in children with learning difficulties. *American Journal of Mental Deficiency, 82,* 559–564.

Carlson, J.S., & Weidl, K.H. (1979). Toward a differential testing approach: Testing-the-limits employing the Raven matrices. *Intelligence, 3,* 323–344.

Collins, J. (1980). Differential treatment in reading groups. In J. Cook-Gumperz (Ed.), *Educational discourse.* London: Heinemann.

Collins, A., Brown, J.S., & Newman, S.E. (in press). Cognitive apprenticeship: Teaching the craft of reading, writing, and mathematics. In L.B. Resnick (Ed.), *Cognition and instruction: Issues and agendas.* Hillsdale, NJ: Erlbaum.

Day, J.D. (1986). Teaching summarization skills: Influences of student ability level and strategy difficulty. *Cognition and Instruction, 3,* 193–210.

Embretson, S.E. (1987). Improving the measurement of spatial aptitude by dynamic testing. *Intelligence, 11,* 333–358.

Erlwanger, S.H. (1973). Benny's conception of rules and answers in IPI mathematics. *Journal of Children's Mathematical Behavior, 1,* 7–26.

Ferrara, R.A. (1987). *Learning mathematics in the zone of proximal development: The importance of flexible use of knowledge.* Unpublished doctoral dissertation, University of Illinois, Champaign.

Ferrara, R.A., Brown, A.L., & Campione, J.C. (1986). Children's learning and transfer of inductive reasoning rules: Studies in proximal development. *Child Development, 57,* 1087–1099.

Feuerstein, R. (1979). *The dynamic assessment of retarded performers: The learning potential assessment device, theory, instruments, and techniques.* Baltimore: University Park Press.

Feuerstein, R. (1980). *Instrumental enrichment: An intervention program for cognitive modifiability.* Baltimore: University Park Press.

Hirsch, E.D., Jr. (1987). *Cultural literacy: What every American needs to know.* Boston: Houghton Mifflin.

Lidz, C.S. (Ed.). (1987). *Dynamic assessment: An interactional approach to evaluating learning potential.* New York: Guilford.

Mehan, H. (1973). Assessing children's language using abilities: Methodological and cross cultural implications. In M. Armer & A.D. Grimshaw (Eds.), *Comparative social research: Methodological problems and strategies* (pp. 309–343). New York: Wiley.

Moore, J., & Newell, A. (1974). How can Merlin understand? In L.W. Gregg (Ed.), *Knowledge and cognition* (pp. 201–252). Hillsdale, NJ: Erlbaum.

Palincsar, A.S., & Brown, A.L. (1984). Reciprocal teaching of comprehension-fostering and monitoring activities. *Cognition and Instruction, 1,* 117–175.

Peck, D.M., Jenks, S.M., & Connell, M.L. (in press). Improving instruction via brief interviews. *Arithmetic Teacher.*

Petitto, A.L. (1985). Division of labor: Procedural learning in teacher-led small groups. *Cognition and Instruction, 2,* 233–270.

Putnam, R.T. (1987). Structuring and adjusting content for students: A study of live and simulated tutoring of addition. *American Educational Research Journal, 24,* 13–48.

Raven, J.C. (1956). *Coloured progressive matrices.* New York: Psychological Corp.

Resnick, L.B. (1982). Syntax and semantics in learning to subtract. In T. Carpenter, J. Moser, & T. Romberg (Eds.), *Addition and subtraction: A cognitive perspective* (pp. 136–158). Hillsdale, NJ: Erlbaum.

Rohwer, W.D., Jr. (1973). Elaboration and learning in childhood and adolescence. In H.W. Reese (Ed.), *Advances in child development and behavior* (Vol. 8, pp. 1–57). New York: Academic Press.

Stodolsky, S. (1988). *The subject matters: Classroom activity in math and social studies.* Chicago: University of Chicago Press.

Vye, N.J., Burns, M.S., Delclos, V.R., & Bransford, J.D. (1987). A comprehensive approach to assessing intellectually handicapped children. In C.S. Lidz (Ed.), *Dynamic assessment: An interactional approach to evaluating learning potential* (pp. 327–359). New York: Guilford.

Vygotsky, L.S. (1978). *Mind in society: The development of higher psychological processes.* (M. Cole, V. John-Steiner, S. Scribner, & E. Souberman, Eds. and Trans.). Cambridge, MA: Harvard University Press.

Wechsler, D. (1974). *Wechsler intelligence scales for children–Revised.* New York: Psychological Corp.

10. Concluding Comments

JOSEPH K. TORGESEN

In these concluding comments, I will summarize the important contributions of the symposium and indicate gaps in our knowledge that were identified in our discussions. I also hope that, by placing ideas from individual authors in a broader context, these comments might stimulate closer study of contributions from individual chapters that may have been overlooked upon first reading.

One of the most important issues on which we focused during our discussions of individual chapters involved the issue of specificity of impairment in children with learning disabilities. As Stanovich pointed out in the first chapter, one of the most fundamental assumptions of our field is that learning disabilities are the result of *specific* impairments in cognitive functioning. These impairments are assumed to affect a limited range of academic (or social) tasks, but do not have a pervasive influence on general intellectual level. This assumption has been under attack in recent years because children with learning disabilities in public school programs have been shown to be similar in their patterns of intellectual abilities to children who perform poorly in school for other reasons (Ysseldyke, Algozzine, Shinn, & McGue, 1982).

Given the fundamental nature of the assumption of specificity, it seems reasonable that a symposium titled "The Cognitive and Behavioral Characteristics of Children with Learning Disabilities" should deal directly with the issue. In fact, much of our discussion considered the question of whether there was, indeed, good research evidence for specific cognitive impairment in children with learning disabilities. We did find evidence in support of the assumption of specificity, but we also identified several reasons why it is frequently difficult to demonstrate specific impairment in random samples of children with learning disabilities who have been in school for any appreciable length of time.

Before I summarize the evidence that led to these conclusions, I should first point out that most of our discussion of specific impairments focused on children whose primary learning disability involved the acquisition of reading skill. Therefore, my summary comments in this area will apply most directly to the problem of reading disabilities. However, our discussion of reasons for the apparent generalized performance deficits of many children with learning disabilities could easily apply to disabilities other than those involving reading.

Evidence for Specific Impairment

Four of the chapters presented either empirical evidence or theoretical discussions concerning the role of phonological processing disabilities as a specific impairment underlying reading disabilities. Stanovich's chapter was the most comprehensive in this regard. The Phonological-Core Variable-Difference Model suggests that problems in processing the phonological features of language are the basic cause of most reading disabilities. This type of disability has its primary effects in limiting the acquisition of fluent decoding skills, and it is not highly correlated with general intellectual level. One general contribution of the mode is that it makes several specific predictions about ways that the cognitive skills of children with specific reading disabilities are employed differently during reading from those of "garden-variety" poor readers. A further important contribution of Stanovich's chapter is his demonstration that, although phonological skills may vary in a continuous fashion among children, it is nevertheless appropriate to single out children with extreme difficulties in this area as specially "handicapped" with regard to reading acquisition.

Chapter 3 (Torgesen) showed how severe phonological processing problems (measured by children's inability to code phonological information in working memory) have a specific impact on reading, as opposed to math, skills. I also showed that the memory impairment of children with phonological coding difficulties was specific to tasks requiring brief, verbatim retention of verbal information. Tasks involving retention of large amounts of meaningfully organized material were not affected. My work also suggests that the phonological processing problems experienced by some children with learning disabilities are an enduring feature of their cognitive system. This supports the idea that such limitations could have a permanent impact on how well these children are able to perform certain types of reading skills.

Felton and Wood (Chapter 5) provided evidence that phonological processing difficulties are characteristic of children with specific reading disabilities as early as the end of first grade. The overall pattern of their results showed that children with reading disabilities could be differentiated from those with broad attentional problems by the specific nature of their impairments on phonological processing tasks. This study was particularly powerful in that it involved a very large sample of randomly selected students, and thus is not subject to many of the sample bias problems of other research on learning disabilities. Finally, although their paper did not focus on the causal, and specific, nature of the relationship between phonological processing problems and reading, Mann, Cowin, and Schoenheimer (Chapter 4) clearly assumed such a relationship and provided ample evidence for it in their introductory comments.

Let us assume, for a moment, that these four chapters are correct in identifying phonological processing problems as a primary characteristic of children with reading disabilities (see more complete discussions in Liberman, 1987; Stanovich, 1986a; Wagner & Torgesen, 1987). Let us also assume that phonological processing difficulties have a specific impact on a limited range of intellectual tasks. Why, then, are there so many challenges to the assumption of specificity in the research literature? Why do children with reading disabilities often appear to be deficient on so many different tasks when compared to children who learn normally? There are at least two possible answers to these questions. First, perhaps phonological processing problems, through their direct effects on higher level language processing tasks, do have a broader effect on cognition than might initially appear to be the case. Second, reading failure itself may have broad consequences for cognitive and behavioral development in young children. Thus, many important characteristics of children with reading disabilities may be thought of as *consequences* of poor reading, rather than as causes of it.

REASONS FOR PERVASIVE COGNITIVE AND BEHAVIORAL IMPAIRMENT

The first possibility, that phonological processing deficits may affect more complex language skills, was directly addressed in the chapter by Virginia Mann and her colleagues. They sought to show how limitations in the ability to store phonological information in working memory can affect children's ability to comprehend the meaning of certain types of sentences. Although we shall see how phonological problems might affect language comprehension indirectly through their effects on reading acquisition, Mann's hypothesis is that they also can have a direct impact because they place limits on the ability of children to process sentences that have complex structure. However, the actual significance of this limitation in the day-to-day language comprehension activities of children with reading disabilities was questioned by Torgesen. He showed that children with learning disabilities who have severe phonological coding problems could comprehend normally organized paragraph and story length material as well as normally achieving children. He did agree, however, that phonological coding disabilities do place limits on "comprehension" of language that must be remembered verbatim, such as strings of orally given directions. At present, the extent to which phonological processing difficulties directly limit the everyday information processing efficiency of children with reading disabilities remains open. It is obviously an area in need of more research.

Three of the chapters contributed information concerning the potential effects of reading failure itself on cognitive and behavioral development in children with learning disabilities (either phonological or otherwise). These effects might be broadly grouped into two areas: effects on general background knowledge, and effects on learning behaviors and attitudes. There can be little doubt that children with reading disabilities have fewer opportunities to acquire information in school than children who read normally (Stanovich, 1986b). Steve Ceci and Jacquelyn Baker provided many illustrations of ways the performance problems of children with learning disabilities might be caused by poorly elaborated knowledge representations. Their work provides extensive verification that the efficiency of many processing operations is affected by the organization and richness of the knowledge base within which they function. Such skills as analogical reasoning, comprehension of discourse, and various kinds of problem solving are all directly affected by both the declarative and procedural knowledge a child possesses. Thus, many kinds of performance deficiencies in children with learning disabilities could be the result of limitations in their knowledge base, which are, in turn, the result of their more basic failure to acquire efficient reading skills.

Dale Schunk and James McKinney provided evidence about possible negative effects of reading disabilities on the development of efficient learning behaviors and attitudes. In his detailed analysis, Schunk showed how consistent failure on important school tasks can lead to a lowered sense of self-efficacy for learning. Low self-efficacy, in turn, is predictive of a lack of persistence on new learning tasks. Thus, his analysis shows how early failure in reading might lead to a set of attitudes and behavior that further limits children's ability to profit from school instruction. His analysis is consistent with other work (Kistner & Torgesen, 1987) indicating the broad effects that early failure can have on the development of both efficient strategies and motivation for school learning in young children. McKinney's more comprehensive analyses of the effects of learning disabilities on behavior showed that many children with learning disabilities who exhibited normal behavior patterns in first grade had been placed in groups with maladaptive behavior patterns by the time they were in third grade. His data also showed that children with learning disabilities and behavioral problems fall increasingly behind their nondisabled peers in achievement with each succeeding school year.

From these latter three chapters, it is clear that one reason that children with learning disabilities may appear to have mild but pervasive cognitive limitations is the emergence of characteristics that must be considered *secondary* to their basic reading failure. These characteristics are consequences of reading disability, rather than causes of it. However, as our discussions suggested, these secondary characteristics are not less important for understanding children with reading disabilities than primary, or specific, characteristics. Once acquired, they can act *causally* in further limiting the child's ability to acquire new information and skills.

In fact, one intriguing possibility suggested by several long-term follow-up studies (Horn, O'Donnell, & Vitulano, 1983) is that effective special education for children with severe reading disabilities may have its major impact on these secondary characteristics, while the primary, and specific, disability is less affected. The long-term findings suggesting this possibility are that children with reading disabilities who receive intensive remedial intervention often can make quite successful adjustments to adult life in spite of retaining a slow and labored reading style resulting from enduring decoding difficulties.

IMPORTANT QUALIFICATIONS

As with any attempt to integrate the contributions of such a diverse and rich group of chapters as those from this symposium, the foregoing discussion leaves a number of important points unaddressed. The first that should be mentioned is the clear possibility that phonological processing difficulties are probably not the only specific cause of reading disabilities. As Stanovich suggested, subtle disabilities in visual/orthographic processing may also contribute to difficulties in acquiring fluent decoding skills in reading. However, there was general agreement that, at present, phonological processing disabilities are the best candidate for a specific processing dysfunction underlying reading disabilities.

The foregoing discussion also did not do justice to a difference in emphasis between the chapter by Ceci and Baker and many of the others. Ceci and Baker preferred to think of limitations in the knowledge base of children with learning disabilities as arising from possible differences in learning opportunities, or experience, rather than resulting from enduring processing limitations. They argued that any inherent, or innate, processing disability would have effects on cognitive development that would be too general to fit the assumption of specificity. However, others argued that one of the strengths of phonological processing disabilities as a candidate for a specific cause of reading disabilities was the potential isolation of its consequences to acquisition of decoding skills. In other words, both data and theory suggest that children might have an enduring, inherent limitation in this area without experiencing direct effects from it in other important areas of cognitive functioning.

Finally, although I earlier discussed behavioral difficulties as secondary characteristics of children with learning disabilities, both McKinney (Chapter 6) and Felton and Wood (Chapter 5) presented data suggesting that a number of very young children with learning disabilities may bring to school a set of behaviors that are maladaptive for classroom learning. In McKinney's work, 65% of the sample of young children with learning disabilities were classified as exhibiting some form of behavioral difficulty that might potentially interfere with classroom learning. In Felton and Wood's study, children with reading disabilities in first grade received higher teacher ratings for attention deficit disorder than did normally achieving children. Both of these findings suggest that, from a very early age, many children with learning disabilities exhibit a complex picture of both cognitive and behavioral differences that can affect their academic performance.

AREAS FOR FUTURE RESEARCH

One of the points on which everyone agreed is that there is still a great deal to be learned about specific learning disabilities! Each author proposed a number of unresolved issues in his or her own area, but several more general research questions also evolved from our discussions. One of the most prominent of these involved the need for more longitudinal research on the development of children with learning disabilities. This method would help to answer important questions in at least three areas. First, it would provide information about the way that the specific, or primary, characteristics of children with learning disabilities develop. One important question with regard to the development of phonological processing skills, for example, is whether individual differences in these skills remain stable over extended periods of time. Second, longitudinal research can help to answer questions about causal relationships between specific processing skills and academic achievement. For example, in order to be considered a causal disability, a given characteristic must be clearly observable *before* an academic deficit emerges, as well as predictive of it. Third, longitudinal research might help us learn more about the relationships among primary, or causal, determinants of learning disabilities, and the secondary characteristics that emerge as a result of academic failure. For example, we clearly need to know more about the emergence of acquired knowledge deficits and maladaptive learning behaviors as they impact on the ability to acquire new knowledge and adapt to new situations.

Joseph Campione's chapter on dynamic assessment proposed a research agenda and methodology that should contribute significantly to our understanding of the ways that the secondary, or acquired, characteristics of children with reading disabilities interfere with their ability to adapt to new learning challenges. If these children suffer an acquired knowledge deficit because of their inability to learn from text, dynamic assessment procedures can potentially provide a fairer opportunity for them to demonstrate their intact cognitive skills. In addition, by focusing on the processes of learning, rather than products, dynamic assessment should provide a clearer picture of possible maladaptive learning styles, or specific knowledge deficits, that hinder academic performance in many children with learning disabilities.

Finally, we must continue to address the basic assumption of specificity through research to identify other potential causes of academic failure that have a focused, limited impact on general intellectual development. Not only must we clearly specify these processing deficits in a set of converging experimental operations, but we must also have good empirical and theoretical evidence that they are, indeed, causal determinants of specific kinds of academic failure. It is not enough simply to show that children with learning disabilities possess a given characteristic; we must also be able to generate convincing theoretical arguments (supported by good experimental evidence) that the effects of the processing disability are limited in scope, but powerful enough to cause meaningful academic impairment on specific tasks.

REFERENCES

Horn, W.F., O'Donnell, J.P., & Vitulano, L.A. (1983). Long-term follow-up studies of learning disabled persons. *Journal of Learning Disabilities, 16,* 542–555.

Kistner, J., & Torgesen, J.K. (1987). Motivational and cognitive aspects of learning disabilities. In A.E. Kasdin & B.B. Lahey (Eds.), *Advances in clinical child psychology* (pp. 289–334). New York: Plenum.

Liberman, I.Y. (1987). Language and literacy: The obligation of the schools of education. In R.F. Bowler (Ed.), *Intimacy with language* (pp. 1–9). Baltimore: The Orton Dyslexia Society.

Stanovich, K.E. (1986a). Explaining the variance in reading ability in terms of psychological processes: What have we learned? *Annals of Dyslexia, 35,* 67–96.

Stanovich, K.E. (1986b). Matthew effects in reading: Some consequences of individual differences in the acquisition of literacy. *Reading Research Quarterly, 21,* 360–406.

Wagner, R.K., & Torgesen, J.K. (1987). The nature of phonological processing and its causal role in the acquisition of reading skills. *Psychological Bulletin, 101,* 192–212.

Ysseldyke, J.E., Algozzine, B., Shinn, M., & McGue, M. (1982). Similarities and differences between underachievers and students labeled learning disabled. *The Journal of Special Education, 16,* 73–85.

About the Authors

Jacquelyn G. Baker is a graduate student at Cornell and has published seven articles and chapters on the topic of learning disabilities. Recently, she received the Creativity Research Fund's dissertation award for her work on individual differences in processing and their relationship to creativity.

Joseph C. Campione is professor of education and director of the Graduate Group in Special Education at the University of California at Berkeley. His interests are in theories of children's learning and transfer performance and the implications of those theories for assessment and instruction.

Stephen J. Ceci is a professor of developmental psychology at Cornell University. He received his PhD from the University of Exeter in 1978 and has been at the Department of Human Development at Cornell since 1980. He is the recipient of the National Institute of Health's Research Career Development Award and a member of five editorial boards. He is a fellow of three divisions of the American Psychological Association and received several awards from that organization. He has published approximately 75 articles, chapters, and commentaries as well as four edited volumes and a single-authored book.

Elizabeth Cowin graduated from Bryn Mawr College with honors in experimental psychology and is currently a graduate student in the Department of Psychology at the University of Toledo.

Rebecca H. Felton, PhD, is assistant research professor in the Section of Neuropsychology, Department of Neurology, Bowman Gray School of Medicine. She received her doctoral degree in child development

221

and learning disabilities from the University of North Carolina at Greensboro. Her major research interests include language and attentional mechanisms in learning disabilities as well as early identification and teaching methods for children at risk for learning disabilities.

Virginia A. Mann is an associate professor in the Department of Cognitive Science at the University of California, Irvine. She received her PhD in experimental psychology in 1977 from the Department of Psychology at MIT. Her research interests focus on developmental issues and presently concern two areas of language development: reading ability and the perception of speech. She has been a research associate at Haskins Laboratories since 1978.

James D. McKinney, PhD, is a professor of education and research professor at the Frank Porter Graham Child Development Center, University of North Carolina at Chapel Hill. He directs the Carolina Learning Disabilities Research Project at the FPG Center.

Joyce Schoenheimer graduated from Bryn Mawr College with honors in experimental psychology and is a graduate student at the City University of New York.

Dale H. Schunk, PhD, is an associate professor of educational psychology, School of Education, University of North Carolina–Chapel Hill. He received his doctoral degree in educational psychology in 1979 from Stanford University. His research specializations are in the areas of social cognitive learning, modeling processes, and motivation.

Keith E. Stanovich received his PhD from the Department of Psychology, University of Michigan; and is currently professor of psychology and education, Oakland University, Rochester, Michigan. He is the associate editor of the journal *Merrill-Palmer Quarterly*. His research interests are in the psychology of reading, reading disabilities, educational psychology, cognitive development, and information processing.

Joseph K. Torgesen is a professor of psychology at Florida State University. He received his PhD from the University of Michigan in 1976. His research interests include the study of memory skills in children with LD and the use of computer-aided practice to enhance basic reading skills in children with reading disabilities. He is the editor, with Bernice Wong, of a recent book titled *Psychological and Educational*

Perspectives on Learning Disabilities and serves on the editorial board of numerous journals.

Frank B. Wood, PhD, is associate professor of Neurology and Psychiatry and section head of the Section of Neuropsychology, Department of Neurology, Bowman Gray School of Medicine. He received his doctoral degree in psychology from Duke University. His major research interests include theoretical neuropsychology, learning disabilities, memory, and the neuropsychology of psychopathology.

Author Index

225

Subject Index

Page numbers in italics refer to figures. Page numbers followed by a "t" refer to tables.